ELECTROACOUSTIC ANALYSIS AND ENHANCEMENT OF ALARYNGEAL SPEECH

ELECTROACOUSTIC ANALYSIS AND ENHANCEMENT OF ALARYNGEAL SPEECH

Edited by

ANDREW SEKEY, Ph.D.

Department of Electrical and Computer Engineering
Computer Systems Laboratory
University of California
Santa Barbara, California

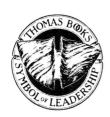

CHARLES C THOMAS • PUBLISHER
Springfield • Illinois • U.S.A.

Published and Distributed Throughout the World by
CHARLES C THOMAS • PUBLISHER
2600 South First Street
Springfield, Illinois, 62703 U.S.A.

© *1982 by* CHARLES C THOMAS • PUBLISHER
ISBN 0-398-04547-X
Library of Congress Catalog Card Number: 81-9082

*With THOMAS BOOKS careful attention is given to all details of
manufacturing and design. It is the Publisher's desire to present books that are
satisfactory as to their physical qualities and artistic possibilities and appropriate for their particular use. THOMAS BOOKS will be true to those laws of
quality that assure a good name and good will.*

Library of Congress Cataloging in Publication Data

Main entry under title:

Electroacoustic analysis and enhancement of alaryngeal speech.

Based upon an interdisciplinary conference held on June 26-27, 1980 at the
University of California, Santa Barbara.
Bibliography: p.
Includes index.
1. Speech, Alaryngeal—Congresses. 2. Electro-acoustics—Congresses. 3. Ar-
tificial larynx—Congresses. 4. Laryngoplasty—Congresses. I. Sekey, Andrew.
RF540.E36   617'.53301   81-9082
ISBN 0-398-04547-X   AACR2

Printed in the United States of America
PS-R-1

CONTRIBUTORS

J. BACH ANDERSEN, dr. techn.
 Institute of Electronic Systems
 Aalborg University Centre
 Aalborg, Denmark

BYRON J. BAILEY, M.D.
 Department of Otolaryngology
 University of Texas Medical Branch
 Galveston, Texas

PETER BRANDERUD, M.Sc.
 Institute of Linguistics
 University of Stockholm
 Stockholm, Sweden

ROBERT L. EVERETT, Ph.D.
 Department of Electrical Engineering
 University of Houston
 Houston, Texas

KAROLY GALYAS, M.Sc.
 Department of Speech Communication
 Royal Institute of Technology (KTH)
 Stockholm, Sweden

LEWIS P. GOLDSTEIN, Ph.D.
 Speech Pathologist
 Veterans Administration Medical Center
 Gainesville, Florida

WILBUR JAMES GOULD, M.D.
 Department of Otolaryngology
 Lenox Hill Hospital
 New York, New York

CERI M. GRIFFITHS, M.D.
Bay Area Ear, Nose & Throat Associates
Houston, Texas

ROBERT HANSON, Ph.D.
Bell Laboratories
Murray Hill, New Jersey

DAVID E. HARTMAN, Ph.D., CCC-SP
Department of Neurology
Gundersen Clinic Ltd.
La Crosse, Wisconsin

YOSHIYUKI HORII, Ph.D.
Department of Communication Disorders
  and Speech Science
University of Colorado
Boulder, Colorado

SATOSHI IMAIZUMI, Ph.D.
Department of Otolaryngology
Kinki University
School of Medicine
Minami-Kawachi-gun
Osaka, Japan

YASUO KOIKE, M.D.
Department of Otolaryngology
Kinki University
School of Medicine
Minami-Kawachi-gun
Osaka, Japan

BJARNE LANGVAD, B.Sc.
Institute of Electronic Systems
Aalborg University Centre
Aalborg, Denmark

BRUCE LEIPZIG, M.D.
Department of Otolaryngology
University of Texas Medical Branch
Galveston, Texas

ROBERT McALLISTER, Ph.D.
  Institute of Linguistics
  University of Stockholm
  Stockholm, Sweden

HENRIK MØLLER, B.Sc.
  Institute of Electronic Systems
  Aalborg University Centre
  Aalborg, Denmark

TOSHIO MONJU, M.D.
  Department of Otolaryngology
  Kinki University
  School of Medicine
  Minami-Kawachi-gun
  Osaka, Japan

THOMAS MURRY, Ph.D.
  Audiology and Speech Pathology
  Veterans Administration Hospital
  San Diego, California

BRUCE W. PEARSON, M.D., F.R.C.S. (C)
  Department of Otolaryngology
  Mayo Clinic
  Rochester, Minnesota

OVE ROLD
  Nordjyllands Amts Taleininstitut
  Aalborg, Denmark

HOWARD B. ROTHMAN, Ph.D.
  Speech Department
  Institute for Advanced Study of the
    Communication Processes
  University of Florida
  Gainesville, Florida

ANDREW SEKEY, Ph.D.
  Department of Electrical and Computer
    Engineering

Computer Systems Laboratory
University of California
Santa Barbara, California

SADANAND SINGH, Ph.D.
  Department of Speech
  California State University
  San Diego, California

ROB C. VAN GEEL, Drs.
  Fonetisch Instituut
  University of Utrecht
  Utrecht, Netherlands

BERND WEINBERG, Ph.D.
  Department of Audiology and
    Speech Sciences
  Purdue University
  West Lafayette, Indiana

ROBERT D. WOODS, II, M.D.
  Otolaryngologist
  Lexington, Kentucky

INTRODUCTION

In the evolution of science and technology every so often a constellation of circumstances occurs at which rapid progress in a specific problem area becomes both necessary and possible. Rehabilitation of laryngectomees has, I believe, arrived at such a juncture. On the sociomedical side, we are looking at an estimated 40,000 laryngectomees in the United States, of whom some 25,000 have undergone total laryngectomy, while about 10,000 new cases of laryngeal cancer are being detected every year. With the increasing average age of the U.S. population, these numbers are likely to increase, and the cost of rehabilitation will be borne, indirectly, by the taxpayer. Meanwhile, the nationwide growth in the awareness of the psychological and social problems of the physically handicapped, exemplified by recent legislation and by the establishment of a National Institute of Handicapped Research, has caused a corresponding rise in the expectations of the disabled population.

Concurrently, we have been witnessing during the past two decades a spectacular growth of activity in computer- and microprocessor-assisted speech science and technology. The once ubiquitous Sonagraph® is gradually being replaced by the evermore sophisticated computer analysis systems. Simultaneous acoustic, electromyographic, palatographic, and other measurements are yielding valuable data on normal as well as pathological speech production. Synthetic speech, until recently only a laboratory curiosity, is finding its way into calculators, clocks, even children's toys.

Lastly, the medical profession, too, is advancing its stance on several fronts. Surgical procedures are becoming more conservative, with refined techniques evolved to delineate cancer-affected tissue. Partial and subtotal laryngectomies are now often performed when in the past the entire larynx would have been removed. New surgical procedures have been invented, such as

ix

the Asai operation or the Staffieri technique, to create a substitute "glottis" for the laryngectomee. Elsewhere, surgical-engineering collaboration is rapidly bringing closer the day of the first human speaking with an implanted artificial larynx.

Such thoughts led me a year ago to propose the first interdisciplinary conference on Electroacoustic Analysis and Enhancement of Laryngectomee Speech. I felt that by offering a forum at which voice scientists, surgeons, electronic engineers, speech pathologists, instrument manufacturers, and laryngectomees themselves could interact, we could provide a catalyst for the hoped-for process of rapid and dramatic progress in the area of laryngectomee rehabilitation.

The conference took place at the University of California, Santa Barbara, on June 26-27, 1980. The audience included representatives of all the above-mentioned disciplines as well as graduate students from the University of California. Though not originally planned as such, the meeting turned out to be fairly international, with five foreign countries represented in addition to the United States.

Of the twenty-six papers presented during the five sessions of the conference, fifteen were invited for inclusion (mostly in a revised form) in this book. The selection was made by an editorial committee guided by the following criteria: papers in this volume had to contain largely previously unpublished material, either original research or reviews with a viewpoint, scope, and critical depth not found in other sources. They also had to be germane to the central theme reflected by the title of the conference and of this volume. An exception was made, however, for the three surgical papers that, while addressing themselves to the enhancement of alaryngeal speech through conservative or reconstructive surgery, do not directly interface with electroacoustics. Our purpose in including them was to provide the anticipated, chiefly nonmedical readership of this volume with relatively popular expositions of techniques leading to the anatomical boundary conditions under which rehabilitative procedures must be performed.

Abstracts of papers presented at the conference but not included in this volume are reproduced in the Appendix, with addresses given of authors from whom complete versions of their paper can be requested.

Readers may be interested in the procedure by which all conference papers were reviewed. Manuscripts received about a month before the conference were sent out to referees, all of whom were registered participants at the conference. Reviewers were asked to identify themselves to their authors at the meeting so as to negotiate any recommended changes. We were gratified to see how many reviewers were actually willing to do so, thus greatly contributing to the friendly, workshop-like exchange of ideas.

Papers in this book are grouped in three parts. Part I, *Analysis and Evaluation of Alaryngeal Speech,* leads off with Weinberg's review of acoustic and temporal characteristics of esophageal speech, the longest chapter in this volume. After a brief summary of prosthetic and surgical rehabilitative techniques, Weinberg illuminates the characteristics of alaryngeal speech from several angles. The chapter by Horii is a good example of new analysis opportunities available to the computer user, in this instance for the measurement of oronasal airflow and fo variations. The point is further buttressed by Imaizumi et al., who applied inverse filtering to (Japanese) speech sounds produced by four different kinds of laryngectomee, for the extraction of the residue waveform and glottal volume velocity. Since the production of the "right" excitation signal, addressed by several other papers in this collection, is one of the core issues of any voice prosthesis, their method will no doubt be of general interest. Neck-type artificial larynges is the topic of Rothman's richly illustrated survey. Besides addressing himself to what makes artificial electronic speech good (or bad), he also deals with the important subject of tissue coupling of neck-type devices. The last chapter in this section by Murry and Singh uses multidimensional scaling to obtain perceptual correlates to physiological and acoustic features of carcinogenic voice.

Part II, *Electroacoustic Speech Aids,* contains seven chapters on a variety of prosthetic devices. This section is led off by Goldstein's survey of many external and internal pneumatic aids, in addition to several electrical ones. Next is a report by Sekey and Hanson on a complex speech-support system currently under development. Two major issues addressed by them—artificial intonation and the excitation of the vocal tract at a point other than the larynx—are also taken up by subsequent chapters.

Specifically, Galyas et al., describe a manual control device for variable pitch, while van Geel advocates a stylized intonation contour, preprogramed but manually triggered. The chapter by Bach Andersen et al., tells of their search for a good excitation waveform for an intraoral device, a problem whose significance has only been recently recognized. The chapter by Galyas and Branderud recommends objective methods for testing the quality of speech amplifiers, clearly an important practical matter for anyone dealing with pathologically weak voices. The section closes with the extensive report by Everett and Bailey on the Texas implanted electrolarynx; it is also a mini-survey by the only U.S. group working on this type of device.

At the panel session held at the end of the conference several significant remarks were made about the contents of this part. One was that, as scientists, we often tend to be overly concerned about the vocal quality of prosthetic aids and pay less attention to such factors as acceptability to the patient, as well as to the speech pathologist community, and the ability of the user population to learn the often rather subtle manipulations required to operate sophisticated devices. Several speakers, especially representatives of manufacturers, stressed the disappointingly poor care some of these instruments receive in the hands of their users. The latter also stressed the small return on large investment for the development and marketing of electrolarynges and the need for university/industry collaborative research grants in this area.

These seem serious matters for consideration by anyone wishing to build a better electrolarynx. Yet I strongly feel that we, writers and readers of this volume, would fail in our task if we allowed the day to come when cheap children's toys would speak good English, while our laryngectomized fellow humans still could not.

Part III, *Surgical-Enhancement Methods,* is an attempt towards closing the gap between the medical and engineering approaches for achieving the same goal. Representatives of two eminent groups in the United States, the University of Texas Medical Branch in Galveston and the Mayo Clinic, have presented three state-of-the-art papers on conservative and reconstructive surgical techniques. Not feeling qualified to comment on these, I invited Dr. Wilbur James Gould to do so, and his remarks appear following Chapter 15.

On the matter of interfacing between engineers and surgeons, Dr. Weinberg suggested during the panel discussion how beneficial it could be if surgeons preparing for the creation of an air by-pass into the vocal tract would be aided by engineers and voice scientists in designing the kind of structure that would behave in a desired way to serve as a voicing source. We have not yet attained this level of symbiosis, but judging by the enthusiasm and collaborative spirit of surgeons participating at the conference, the willingness is there.

In closing, it is my pleasure to acknowledge the many professional colleagues who have contributed to this enterprise. First, much credit for assistance in various phases of organization is due my colleague and cochairman of the conference, Robert Hanson, whose departure from UC Santa Barbara prevented him from participating in the task of editing. I am grateful to Lewis Goldstein, Howard Rothman, and Bernd Weinberg who, as members of the editorial committee, shared with Bob Hanson and myself the responsibility of selecting the papers for this volume. Likewise, thanks are due to the session chairmen, Krzysztof Izdebski, Thomas Murry, Colin Painter, Howard Rothman, and John Snidecor. (The last-mentioned "elder statesman" of the scientific study of laryngectomee speech, and to our fortune a very accessible professor emeritus at our university, also freely offered his counsel on various matters relating to the conference.)

Funding for the conference was provided by a grant from the University of California Cancer Research Coordinating Committee, and operating losses were underwritten by the associate vice chancellor for research and academic development at UC Santa Barbara. Secretarial chores were cheerfully handled by Suzie Garcia and Catherine Stadem. Finally, collective thanks are due to our graduate students, too numerous to name, who gave their time and dedication thus contributing greatly to the smooth running of the conference.

A.S.

CONTENTS

ELECTROACOUSTIC ANALYSIS
AND ENHANCEMENT
OF ALARYNGEAL SPEECH

PART I:
ANALYSIS AND EVALUATION OF ALARYNGEAL SPEECH

SPEECH AFTER LARYNGECTOMY: AN OVERVIEW AND REVIEW OF ACOUSTIC AND TEMPORAL CHARACTERISTICS OF ESOPHAGEAL SPEECH

BERND WEINBERG

ABSTRACT

In this chapter, a brief review of the mechanisms of alaryngeal speech and voice production is provided. A detailed description of acoustic and temporal characteristics (fundamental frequency, intensity, long and short-time spectra, rate, vocal quality, extraneous sounds) of esophageal speech is provided together with a review of critical anatomical and physiological properties underlying esophageal speech/voice production. Particular emphasis is also directed toward explicating linguistic aspects of speech after laryngectomy. Information is interpreted to (1) provide insights about the precise nature of the impact occasioned by larynx removal on speech; (2) identify areas of information scarcity, and (3) highlight the role that studies of laryngectomized patients may play in solving important questions about speech production/perception in general.

INTRODUCTION

SURGICAL REMOVAL OF THE larynx is a procedure often performed on patients with laryngeal cancer. Total laryngectomy neccessitates removal of the entire laryngeal framework. In this procedure, all structures located between the hyoid bone and the upper tracheal rings are sacrificed. The trachea is rotated forward and sutured to a surgically created opening. This leads to the creation of a permanent stoma on the external neck wall for respiratory purposes and results in an anatomical, but not

5

functional, separation between the pulmonary airway and the digestive tract.

Total laryngectomy surgery always results in a sacrifice of tissue essential to normal vocal function and in considerable alteration of the anatomy and physiology of the speech mechanism. As a result, the normal processes of speech are modified to such a great extent that there is always a complete loss of the ability to produce voice by conventional means. Laryngectomized patients compensate for this loss by using alternative methods of voicing to support speech production.

Basically, there are two forms of voicing laryngectomized persons may use to support alaryngeal speech production. One form refers to extrinsic methods of alaryngeal voice and speech. Extrinsic forms depend upon man-made voicing prosthesis (artificial larynges) or surgically created structures developed specifically for the purpose of voice production (surgical/prosthetic approaches to voice restoration). The second form is an intrinsic method that relies upon intrinsic anatomical structures remaining following laryngeal extirpation (e.g. esophageal voice/speech).

EXTRINSIC FORMS OF ALARYNGEAL VOICE AND SPEECH
Artificial Larynges

A common form of alaryngeal speech involves the use of a prosthetic voicing source, or artificial larynx. There are two principal reasons for the widespread and increasing use of artificial larynges: (1) patient preference for the artificial larynx as a primary method of oral communication; and (2) failure of large numbers of laryngectomized patients to attain functionally serviceable esophageal speech.

Although a wide variety of artificial larynges are currently available, clinical or basic research studies concerned with important aspects of artificial larynx usage are scarce. This situation is primarily the result of a long-standing view in which the artificial larynx was regarded as a backup method for patients who failed to achieve esophageal speech (Lauder 1968). This philosophy was popular until about a decade ago when Diedrich argued that a primary goal of alaryngeal speech rehabilitation was to develop functional communication, regardless of the mode of voicing. The Diedrich concept, coupled with the fact that there is no evidence that the use of an artificial larynx reduces the laryngectomized patient's ability to learn esophageal speech, gave rise to increasing interest in the use of artificial larynges as alternative and primary modes of voicing support for speech.

Efficient use of an artificial larynx as a voicing source clearly does not depend on the integrity of the esophagus and the pharynesophageal (P-E) segment. The prosthetic device itself serves as the vibratory source. The voicing source of these devices are powered either by pulmonary air or by electronic means. Stated differently, pneumatic instruments utilize pulmonary air from the stoma to activate a voicing source. Electronic artificial larynges are battery powered and generate a sound into the vocal tract on either a transcervical or intraoral basis. The characteristics of the voice produced by an artificial larynx depend on the acoustic characteristics of the source and the properties of the laryngectomized patient's altered vocal tract.

In an early classic series of papers, Barney (1958) provided information about four important areas related to the development of speech aids: design objectives, acoustic factors that affect speech quality, consonant production, and speech intelligibility. Barney's discussion of these critical areas is lucid, technically sound, and clinically relevant. Barney (1959) has also described the development of the Western Electric Model No. 5 (A and B) artificial larynx. This electronic device is currently the most widely used artificial larynx. Hence, both the historical perspectives and the technical background surrounding its development should be understood. Both articles by Barney should be required reading for all persons involved in speech rehabilitation for laryngectomized patients.

It is generally agreed that desirable attributes of any type of artificial larynx, originally described by Barney (1958), should include:

1. Output speech intensity equal to that of normal speech
2. Output speech quality and prosody comparable to that of normal speech
3. Inconspicuousness
4. Hygienically acceptable to the user

5. Simple to operate
6. Reliability
7. Low cost

Descriptive study and clinical experience indicate that none of the artificial larynges currently available adequately meet all of these design attributes (*see* Bennett and Weinberg 1973; Weinberg and Riekena 1973). Voice produced by most artificial larynges is characterized by a mechanical or electronic quality with limited variation in f_o (pitch) or intensity (loudness) (Barney 1958; Weinberg and Bennett 1973).

A detailed review of properties of speech produced with various types of artificial larynges is provided by Rothman (see Chapter 4). Hence, we will not review this material in this presentation.

Surgical-Prosthetic Methods of Voice/Speech Restoration

An obvious primary postsurgical rehabilitation goal for laryngectomized patients is complete restoration of oral communication. To date, this objective has largely been accomplished using the time-honored method of esophageal speech or through the use of artificial larynges. In recent years the field of alaryngeal speech rehabilitation has experienced a resurgence of interest in developing surgical prosthetic methods of speech/voice restoration. As indicated previously, these methods require laryngectomized patients to effect voicing by relying upon surgically created structures developed specifically for the purpose of voice production. All contemporary methods are characterized by functional liabilities and all have one common feature: the surgical reconnection between the pulmonary airway and the laryngectomized patient's vocal tract or new phonatory apparatus (Shedd and Weinberg 1980). For example, some of these methods seek to develop an air shunt, or connection, between the trachea and the esophagus or between the trachea and the pharynx (Conley, DeAmesti, and Pierce 1958; Miller 1967; Calcaterra and Jafek 1973; Taub and Bergner 1973; Komorn 1974; Sisson et al. 1975; Singer and Blom 1980). Others seek to interpose both an air shunt and a mechanical voicing source between the trachea and pharynx (Weinberg, Shedd, and Horii 1978). Finally, there is a method in which a mechanical voicing source is surgically implanted in the pharynx (Young, Everett, and Barley 1980; Fredrickson 1980).

Most methods of surgical-prosthetic speech restoration involve the surgical creation of a connection between the trachea and esophagus or hypopharynx (Conley, DeAmesti, and Pierce 1958; Calcaterra and Jafek 1973; Miller 1973; Taub and Bergner 1973; Komorn 1974; Sisson et al. 1975). This connection serves as an air shunt that enables laryngectomized patients to power esophageal phonation with pulmonary air (Conley, DeAmesti, and Pierce 1958; Calcaterra and Jafek 1973; Taub and Bergner 1973; Komorn 1974) or to power an unspecified vibratory source with pulmonary air (Miller 1973; Sisson et al. 1975). In view of this situation, speech produced by these methods should not be expected to exceed levels of overall acceptability obtained by highly proficient esophageal speakers. These methods may enable patients to acquire voice and speech more rapidly, since the need to learn esophageal insufflation techniques is eliminated by virtue of their reliance upon pulmonary air.

In contrast to air-shunt methods, the surgical-prosthetic approaches to speech and voice restoration discussed by Vega (1975), by Griffiths and Love (1978), and by Weinberg, Shedd, and Horii (1978) enable laryngectomized patients to power newly formed vibratory sources with pulmonary air. Vega and Griffiths and Love highlight the techniques described by Staffieri. The Staffieri technique has attracted the attention of a number of American surgeons who are currently adopting this method of voice restoration. Basically, this method involves reconstruction of what Staffieri calls a "phonatory neoglottis" as part of total laryngectomy. Although this method has attracted worldwide attention in recent years, readers will soon realize that the belief that the surgically created "neoglottis" serves as a vibratory or voicing source remains undocumented.

Weinberg, Shedd, and Horii (1978) have described the reed-fistula method of speech, a surgical-prosthetic approach to speech rehabilitation for patients who have undergone extensive resection of the pharynx in association with total laryngectomy. The reed-fistula approach consists of interposing an external air bypass and pseudolaryngeal mechanism between the laryngecto-mized patient's tracheal stoma and a surgically created pharyngeal fistula. The pseudolarynx is a modified Tokyo artificial larynx mechanism (Weinberg and Riekena 1973). This method differs from other approaches in that it is modeled on principles of normal speech production. Simply stated, the reed-fistula approach consists of developing an external larynx (voicing source) and incorporating this new mechanism into the patient's highly integrated speech production system.

Simpson, Smith, and Gordon (1972) have described four types of surgical reconstructions of the pharyngoesophageal segment. Speech and surgical specialists have often expressed the view that improvement in the rate and efficiency of voice reacquisition with esophageal phonation might be increased if consideration were given to surgically altering the morphology of the P-E segment following laryngectomy. Simpson, Smith, and Gordon describe just this, and the results of their work should provide thought-provoking information to all readers.

There is a substantial body of information about a variety of surgical-prosthetic approaches to speech and voice restoration. The majority of these reports highlight the surgical-prosthetic techniques used to implement these methods, while the information about the speech characteristics effected is scanty. The observations support the hypothesis that functionally serviceable speech has been provided to some laryngectomized patients by each of these methods. Although this is true, each of the methods is characterized by some relative liabilities.

The amount of information available concerning speech/voice characteristics effected by these methods is scanty and does not permit the formation of conclusions about the relative adequacy of speech effected by these methods to be made.

INTRINSIC FORMS OF ALARYNGEAL VOICE AND SPEECH

Esophageal Voice/Speech

The impact of larynx removal as part of oncologic therapy is pervasive. Total laryngectomy results in radical changes in man's essential physiology, anatomical makeup, social process of communication, and psychosocial interactions. From a communication point of view, esophageal speech is the most widely used form of alaryngeal communication. Hence, the remaining portions of this chapter will be concerned with this important intrinsic form of alaryngeal voice and speech. Particular emphasis is directed toward providing a detailed description of acoustical and temporal characteristics of esophageal speech. Data are interpreted to provide insights about the precise nature of the impact occasioned by larnyx extirpation on speech, to identify areas of information scarcity, and to highlight the role that study of laryngectomized speakers may play in solving important questions about speech production/perception in general.

Esophageal Voicing: General Requirements

Production of esophageal voicing necessitates use of the esophagus as an accessory lung and the pharyngoesophageal (P-E) segment as a voicing source. The P-E segment is the upper sphincter of the esophagus and serves to divide the pharynx from the esophagus. In normal humans, this segment consists of the cricopharyngeus muscle, fibers of the pharyngeal inferior constrictor, and upper fibers of esophageal muscle (Ellis 1971; Zaino et al. 1970). The P-E segment does undergo major morphological and functional change as a result of laryngeal extirpation. Larynx removal results in a significant sacrifice of tissue critical to postsurgical esophageal voice acquisition. Moreover, the morphological and physiological characteristics of the P-E segment in laryngectomized patients are highly variable.

On an oversimplified basis, the production of esophageal voicing can be described as a two-part process: air intake and voicing. The esophageal speaker must cause a pressure drop across the P-E segment to effect either air intake or voicing.

Esophageal speakers insufflate air into the esophagus by means of the injection or the inhalation methods of air intake. The injection method of air intake is a positive pressure respiratory maneuver. Basically, persons using this method complete tongue compression maneuvers and/or articulatory gestures to generate increased oral and pharyngeal pressure. The magnitude of these pressures must be large enough to override pressure in the P-E segment, causing the segment to open and permit air to enter the esophagus. Moolenaar-Bijl (1953), a Dutch speech therapist, provided the original description of what is now known as *consonant injection* and was the first person to advance the notion that esophageal insufflation can occur as a result of pressure build up associated with the production of certain types of consonants. Weinberg and Bosma (1970) have described a second type of injection, now known as *glossal* or *glossopharyngeal press*. In this case, the compression maneuver is a separate act analogous to glossopharyngeal, or frog, breathing.

By contrast, the inhalation method of air intake is a pulmonary activated method of air insufflation. Air is taken into the esophagus synchronously with pulmonary inhalation. In this method, air is directed into the esophagus by having patients inhale pulmonary air, a behavior that causes the magnitude of negative pressure in the esophagus to increase. Patients are instructed either to keep their mouths open or to sniff during pulmonary inhalation. Under these two conditions, air pressure in the mouth will be positive, i.e. roughly equivalent to atmospheric pressure. Hence, air will flow from the area of positive pressure (mouth and pharynx) to the area of the increased negative pressure (esophagus), provided that the resistance of the P-E segment can be overcome.

Following insufflation of air into the esophagus, the speaker must develop a transpseudoglottal pressure differential to drive the P-E segment into oscillation. In this case, the differential pressure relationship is always characterized by esophageal pressures that exceed the resistance offered by the P-E segment. Stated differently, the speaker must develop positive esophageal pressure of sufficient magnitude to exceed the resistance offered by the closed P-E segment, causing the segment to vibrate for voicing.

Anatomical and Physiological Aspects of Esophageal Speech/Voice Production

The current state of knowledge about fundamental aspects of esophageal phonation and speech is limited. For example, information about the anatomical and physiological mechanisms underlying control of fundamental aspects of esophageal phonation is lacking. In addition, studies of anatomical and physiological mechanisms underlying the control of articulatory and linguistic behaviors of esophageal speakers are also lacking.

Early classic investigations in this area attempted to delineate the nature of change in both the structure and the function of the pharynx and the esophagus resulting from laryngectomy. For example, Kirchner et al. (1963) sought answers to these questions in data obtained from cinefluorographic examinations and intraluminal pressure measurements of the pharynx and the esophagus. It is now clear that the points of attachment of a large number of extrinsic laryngeal muscles along with the cricopharyngeus muscle are sacrificed during total laryngectomy surgery. Existing data provide ample support for the notion that the voicing source used to support esophageal speech should be regarded as a surgical residue characterized by extensive inter-subject variability. Moreover, the relationships between speech or vocal proficiency and morphological or physiological character-istics of the P-E segment or esophagus remain unspecified.

The evidence provided by Kirchner et al. (1963), by Diedrich (1968), and by Winans, Riechbach, and Waldrop (1974) suggests that total laryngectomy may lead to only slight alterations in the anatomy and physiology of the esophagus. As stated, laryngeal attachments of the cricopharyngeus muscle are, of necessity, cut when removing the larynx. This may account for the observa-tions of weakened contractions of the cricopharyngeus muscle postsurgery (Kirchner et al. 1963; Winans et al. 1974) and for altered patterns of contraction in the upper esophagus in some laryngectomized patients. The observations of Kirchner et al. reveal that the amplitude of esophageal peristalsis may be depressed in the area of the upper esophagus, but that the function of the lower esophageal sphincter is apparently not altered by disturbances of the function of the upper esophagus or of the cricopharyngeus muscle. The body of the esophagus in laryngectomized patients, like that of normal speakers, is bound-ed at both ends by a zone of elevated pressure, while resting intraesophageal pressure is negative relative to atmospheric pressure.

The P-E segment does undergo major morphological and functional change as result of laryngeal extirpation. The observa-tions of Diedrich, of Kirchner et al., and others reveal that some laryngectomized patients exhibit well-defined, single P-E segments, typically located between cervical vertebrae four and six. In other patients, more than one segment was observed. For example, some patients exhibited double and triple segments. Finally, Diedrich and Youngstrom (1966) failed to observe a well-defined P-E segment during voice production in a small number of esophageal speakers. The high degree of variability in the morphological characteristics of the segment represents a consistent, reasonable, and clinically relevant observation. Such observations serve to verify the heterogeneity in vocal attributes evident across a large sample of esophageal talkers. The observation that the morphology of the P-E segment in laryngectomized patients is highly variable is not surprising, provided the postsurgical characteristics of the segment are regarded as surgical residue.

CHARACTERISTICS OF ESOPHAGEAL SPEECH

Phonatory Characteristics

A large body of research has been conducted to describe some of the important characteristics of esophageal speech. Since total laryngectomy always results in a sacrifice of tissue essential to normal vocal function, clinicians and investigators have assumed that the principal factors influenced by laryngectomy are those related to the voicing source. Hence, there have been a number of studies completed to specify the fundamental frequency (f_0) characteristics of esophageal speech. A review of this information reveals that the fundamental frequency characteristics of esophageal speakers are now well understood. The average f_0 for male esophageal speakers is about 65 Hz, a value approximately one octave below that expected for normal adult speakers. Average f_0 for individual esophageal speakers exhibit extensive variablity—the range in mean f_0 for speakers extends from approximately 30 to 200 Hz (Kytta 1964; Curry and Snidecor 1959, 1960, 1961; Hoops and Noll 1969; Shipp 1967; Damste 1958 and Weinberg and Bennett 1972). Average f_0 characteristics of esophageal speech also differ as a function of speaker sex (Weinberg and Bennett 1972).

Existing data clearly indicate that esophageal speakers are able to phonate over a wide range of fundamental frequencies. On the average, esophageal speakers exhibit f_0 standard deviation values between 4-4.5 semitones and 90 percent ranges of about 13 semitones. The mean rate of fundamental frequency change during inflections for esophageal speakers is reported to be 7.9 tones per second and 17.7 tones per second for normal speakers. During frequency shifts, the reported values are 4.3 and 7.0 tones per second, respectively. The rate of frequency change for superior esophageal speakers was about one-half the value observed in normal speakers (Snidecor and Curry 1959). Although existing data clearly indicate that esophageal speakers are able to phonate over a wide range of fundamental frequencies, the extent to which they are able to exercise intention and systematic control over f_0 is not well understood.

In this context, Angermeier and Weinberg (1980) subjected esophageal and normal speakers to a pitch-matching task to assess the comparative f_0 control capabilities of these two groups of subjects. Control was assessed by two principal measures. For example, the relative accuracy of the pitch matches was evaluated by calculating the difference between the average f_0 of each vowel production and the average f_0 of nearest octave multiple of steady-state targets. The average differences in f_0 between individual targets and productions were comparable for esophageal and normal talkers. In addition, the distributional properties of production f_0 in relation to those of the targets were also plotted. As expected, the distributions of production f_0 for normal speakers were unimodal, relatively narrow. These data confirmed that normal speakers perceived and completed vocal pitch-matching in a steady-state fashion (*see* Figure 1-1).

The data for esophageal speakers were considerably different. The distributional properties of f_0 for this group exhibited extensive inter- and intra-subject variability, were not unimodal, and were relatively wide (*see* Figure 1-2). The frequency variation associated with pitch-matching by esophageal speakers was 1.5 to 8 times greater than that by normal speakers (*see* Figure 1-3).

These results provide confirmatory support for the belief that esophageal speakers are generally far less proficient in con-

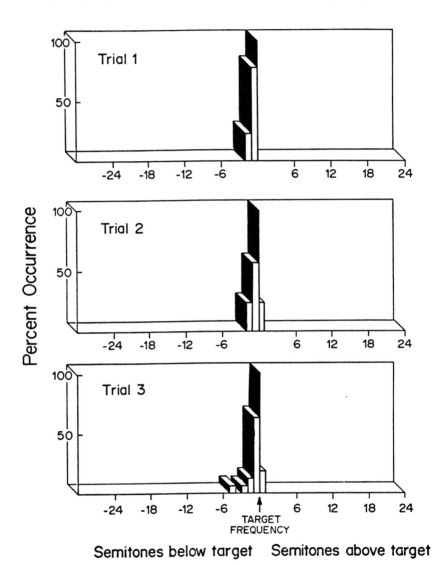

Figure 1-1. Examples of distributions of fundamental frequency associated with vocal pitch-matching by normal speakers. Distributions reflect performance of Speaker 3 in response to 109 Hz target.

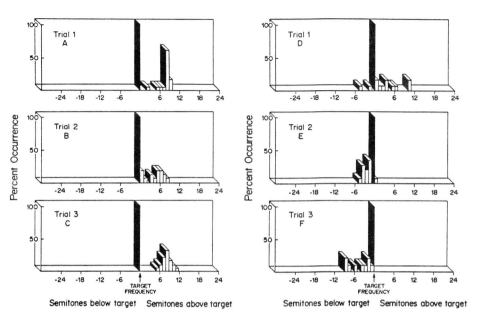

Figure 1-2. Examples of the distributions of fundamental frequency associated with pitch matching by esophageal speakers. Distributions *A-C* summarize performance of Speaker 2 in response to 45 Hz target and reflect the variability in performance and limited manifestation of unimodality (*C*). Distributions *D-F* reflect performance of Speaker 3 in response to 72 Hz target.

trolling steady-state vocal output attributes. Smith et al. (1978) have recently shown that the magnitude of vocal jitter (expressed in either absolute or relative terms) present in sustained vowels produced by esophageal speakers is substantially larger than that observed in comparable utterances produced by normal speakers and speakers with vocal/laryngeal pathologies. They found that the average magnitudes of vocal jitter associated with esophageal voicing ranged between 0.62 and 5.13 msec; standard deviation ranged from 0.44 to 5.18 msec. Average jitter values measured in comparable speech utterances produced by normal speakers ranged between 0.01 and 3.06 msec. These comparative results support the notion of Smith et al. (1978) ". . . that the mechanism esophageal speakers use to control or regulate f_0 is substantially inferior to that employed by normal speakers." Taken together,

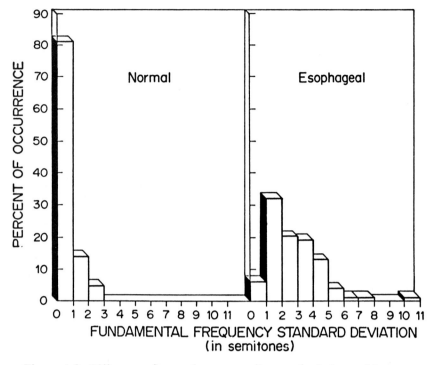

Figure 1-3. Differences in steady-state attributes of pitch-matching performance between normal and esophageal speakers.

the contemporary view is that esophageal speakers exhibit impoverished intentional control over crucial aspects of their vocal output. This view takes cognizance of the marked differences between esophageal and normal voicing source properties.

It is now well established that the production of normal voice is accomplished by a dynamic interplay between respiratory driving forces and laryngeal adjustments. The normal sound source incorporates a set of paired muscle groups that oscillate in a quasi-periodic fashion when driven by pulmonary air. By contrast, the production of voice by esophageal speakers involves using the esophagus as an accessory lung and a surgically reconstructed or residual P-E sphincter as a voicing source. Utilization of the P-E sphincter as a sound source necessitates excitation of an unpaired, fibromuscular structure.

The P-E segment is apparently not supported by an abductor-adductor system, and there is no evidence to support the view that laryngectomized individuals are capable of altering the level of muscular activity within the P-E segment on a systematic basis to control or influence the vibratory rate of this sphincter. Moreover, there is no evidence to suggest that esophageal speakers are able to pretune or systematically adjust the inherent properties of their voicing source for such purposes.

For example, in an electromyographic study of muscular activity of the inferior constrictor and cricopharyngeus in laryngectomized speakers using esophageal speech, Shipp (1970) failed to observe any consistent "typical or modal patterns" of muscle activity, and noted that there was substantial intersubject variation in the patterning of muscular activity of these muscles during voicing. These observations led Shipp to conclude that: "The most noteworthy finding of the muscle activity during the phonatory portion of alaryngeal voice was that no single type of activity emerged as the typical, average, or modal pattern of muscle behavior. The pattern variations obtained were too numerous to classify."

Finally, there are the issues of vocal efficiency and source resistance. Using time-honored experimental techniques, Snidecor and Isshiki have provided the most comprehensive information about airflow and volume characteristics of esophageal speech. One of the more salient findings stemming from their work is the observation of diminished airflow and volume characteristics associated with the production of esophageal voice. For example, the mean flow rate associated with sustained vowels produced by esophageal speakers ranged from about 30-70 cc/sec. These values are markedly lower than those associated with normal vowel production, where flow rates range from about 100-200 cc/sec. These data, coupled with information about esophageal pressures during vowel production, shed light upon the efficacy of the P-E segment as a voicing generator. Specifically, esophageal pressure ranges between about 20-60 cm H_2O during sustained vowel production by esophageal speakers. In this case, the pressure values are markedly higher than those associated with normal vowel production, where subglottic pressure typically ranges between about 3-10 cm H_2O. Taken together, current data suggest that the resistance (pseudoglottal resistance) offered by the voicing source associated with esophageal phonation is an order-of-magnitude larger than that offered by the larynx. Thus, in addition to being a surgical residue devoid of abductor-adductor properties, the voicing source of esophageal speech appears to be a heavily mass-loaded, high-impedance source.

Although it is reasonable to conclude that the fundamental frequency characteristics of esophageal voice are reasonably well understood, information concerning additional salient aspects of esophageal phonation is lacking. For example, the nature of anatomical and physiological mechanisms underlying the regulation of f_o and vocal intensity are not understood. Published data concerning acoustic characteristics of esophageal voice other than f_o, for example, source spectral characteristics, is also not available. Such information is essential to future understanding of quality attributes of esophageal voice and to the development of models or theories of esophageal phonation.

Rate and Temporal Characteristics

It is clear that until recently the majority of research and clinical work dealing with esophageal speech has been directed toward problems associated with voice reacquisition and toward description of selected attributes of esophageal voice. Total laryngectomy surgery also causes substantial changes in the nonphonatory aspects of speech production. For example, Snidecor and Curry (1959, 1960) and others have clearly demonstrated that the speech rate of esophageal speakers is markedly reduced. The speaking rate of superior esophageal speakers ranged from 85 to 129 words per minute, with a group average of 113 words per minute. The assumption has always been that the decrement in rate of esophageal speech is due to the increase in the amount of time these speakers spend in silence. This increase in silent time results from the esophageal speaker's limited ability to sustain voicing. For example, the esophageal speaker produces an average of five words per air charge compared to a mean of 12.5 words per breath group produced by normal speakers (Snidecor and Curry 1959). Hence, the esophageal speaker must pause more often for air intake. In addition, Snidecor and Curry (1960) observed differential length in pauses occurring in the esopha-

geal speech. For example, phrase-limiting pauses (i.e. jʋ
pauses) were approximately 1.41 times longer than ai
pauses. The mean duration of pauses signaling juncture ın
esophageal speech was also greater than the mean duration of
junctural pauses measured for a normal speaker. Finally, it is
possible that articulatory rate, per se, may be altered following
laryngectomy.

Articulation/Intelligibility

Although comprehensive knowledge about articulatory changes
due to laryngeal extirpation is lacking, there is experimental
evidence to support the notion that total laryngectomy surgery
does alter articulatory behavior. For example, the hyoid bone is
often removed during total laryngectomy, and its removal
necessitates disruption of much of the musculature of the
suprahyoid complex and supporting musculature of the tongue.
Such disruptions, coupled with the deprivation of pulmonary
support, are likely to affect the articulatory dynamics of laryngectomized patients. Diedrich (1968) has noted a number of general
changes in articulatory dynamics of esophageal speakers. For
example, esophageal speakers evidenced more continuous movement of the tongue and shorter duration of articulatory contact of
the tongue or lips in comparison with durations sampled on a
preoperative basis in this group of patients. Sisty and Weinberg (1972) have shown that removal of the larynx does alter
vocal-cavity transmission characteristics (*see* Figures 1-4 and 1-5).
The observation that the average vowel formant frequency values
associated with esophageal speech are elevated was interpreted to
support the view that laryngectomized patients exhibit a reduced
vocal tract length. Sacco, Mann, and Schultz (1967), Creech (1966),
and Tikofsky (1965) provide strong support for the general
beliefs that, on the average, esophageal speech is characterized by
a reduction in intelligibility and that efficient contrast of the
voicing (voiced versus voiceless) feature is difficult for esophageal
speakers to achieve. These results lend credence to the view that
extirpation of the larynx results in substantial changes in both
phonatory and nonphonatory aspects of speech production.

Although it is now clear that, on the average, esophageal

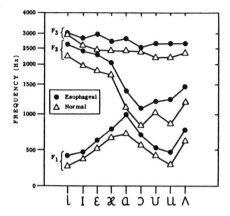

Figure 1-4. Comparison of mean formant frequencies for esophageal and normal male speakers.

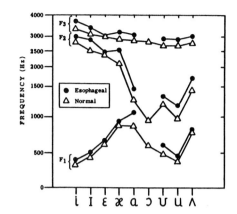

Figure 1-5. Comparison of mean formant frequencies for esophageal and normal female speakers.

speakers exhibit reduced overall intelligibility, the precise nature of the articulatory behaviors employed by esophageal speakers have not been examined on a direct basis. In view of the importance of these behaviors to communication efficacy, this area of research endeavor must receive increased attention.

Unfortunately, the writings of some authors have led some to accept the view that articulatory dynamics of esophageal and normal speakers are comparable. For example, Damste (1958, p. 47) has written: "...The rest of the vocal tract (pharyngeal and oral cavity) behaves substantially the same in normal and esophageal speech." Such statements are highly misleading and not in keeping with contemporary knowledge. The contemporary view is that removal of the larynx results in pervasive changes that influence both the vocal and articulatory substrates of speech. Larynx removal clearly disrupts muscular support to the tongue, occasions major deprivation in respiratory support, and produces alteration in vocal tract morphology. These changes make it apparent that articulatory dynamics of normal and esophageal speakers cannot be comparable. Moreover, the intrusion of gestures for esophageal insufflation of air must exert additional, profound disruptions on co-articulatory constraints and behaviors in laryngectomized speakers using esophageal speech.

Long-Time Intensity and Spectral Characteristics

A major thesis developed in this chapter is that the effects of larynx removal are *pervasive*. An additional parameter of speech influenced by total laryngectomy is *intensity*. We recently assessed the distributional properties of speech intensity of esophageal speakers and compared these characteristics with those of normal speakers (Weinberg, Horii, and Smith 1980). The distributional properties of speech intensity for ten esophageal and five normal speakers are illustrated in Figure 1-6 and reveal substantial differences between intensity characteristics associated with the production of continuous discourse by normal and esophageal talkers.

One such difference is the increased prevalence of lower-level sound output of esophageal compared with normal speech. The modal intensity level is approximately 67 db SPL for the esophageal speakers and 82 db SPL for the normal speakers. In addition, the intensity distribution for normal speech is negatively skewed and reveals a relatively clear difference between speech

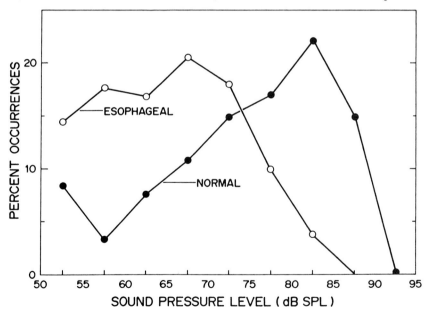

Figure 1-6. Distributional properties of speech intensity.

and pause segments. In contrast, the intensity distribution for esophageal speech is characterized by considerably lower levels and, therefore, less distinction is evident between speech and pause segments. In terms of median intensity levels, there is approximately a 10 db difference between the speech samples of the two groups of talkers.

These data also serve to highlight the relative difference in average intensity between normal and esophageal speech and provide support for the notion that, on the average, esophageal speech is produced at levels of 6-10 db below that typically found for normal speech (Hyman 1955; Snidecor and Isshiki 1965; Hoops and Noll 1969). In passing, it may be noted that total speaking time of esophageal speakers was approximately 55 percent longer than that of the normal speakers. The esophageal speakers spent 23 percent of their time in silence (intensity levels below 50 db SPL), while the normal speakers spent about 14 percent in silence.

As part of the project just described, measurements were also made on long-time spectral characteristics of normal and esophageal speech. Composite average spectra for the two speaker groups are shown in Figure 1-7. For this figure, the maximum level associated with peaks appropriate of F1 energy concentration in the average spectra were used as references (0 db). The composite long-time spectrum of the five normal male speakers was roughly comparable to similar data (derived through filter-bank methods) reported in the literature (Crandall and Mackenzie 1922; Dunn and White 1940; Horii and Hughes 1972; Horii et al. 1973). The average spectrum for esophageal speech was characterized by a flattened spectral envelope, i.e. there was greater relative amplitude in the high-frequency components compared with that measured for normal speech.

The same average spectra of the two groups adjusted for appropriate overall intensity differences are shown in Figure 1-8. The figure shows that the average spectral level of esophageal speech was considerably lower than the normal speech. This was particularly true at two frequency regions: 0-3000 Hz region and 6000-9000 Hz region. The average esophageal spectrum was approximately 10 db lower in the low-frequency region and about 7 db lower around the 6000-9000 Hz region.

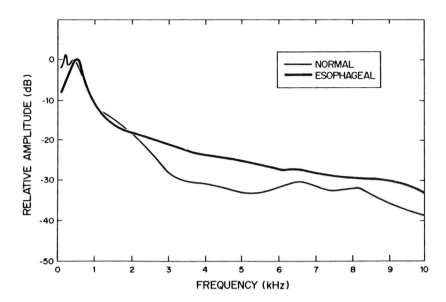

Figure 1-7. Average long-time spectra.

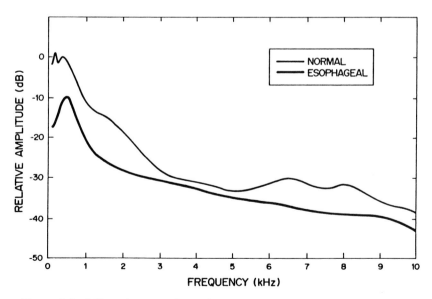

Figure 1-8. Adjusted average long-time spectra.

The lower-frequency region represents primarily vocalic sounds such as vowels, semi-vowels, nasals, and liquids, while the high-frequency region reflects predominantly consonantal sounds such as fricatives, affricates, and stops. Examination of individual average spectra revealed that a spectral maximum (except the fundamental frequency components) was located around 300-450 Hz for normal speakers and between 425-500 Hz for esophageal speakers. These peaks or maxima appear to represent the average first formant frequencies of the vocalic sounds. Sisty and Weinberg (1972) reported increased average vowel formant frequencies in esophageal speech and attributed the finding to shortened overall vocal-tract length caused by the position of neoglottis in esophageal speakers.

Between 1400 Hz and 3000 Hz, the spectral slope associated with the production of normal speech was approximately –10 db/octave. This value is in close agreement with slope data reported by Dunn and White (1940). On the other hand, the slope for esophageal speech in the same frequency region was approximately –3 db/octave. This attenuation in slope may indicate that the amplitudes of higher harmonics associated with esophageal voicing may decrease more slowly than those associated with normal laryngeal voicing. This, in turn, suggests more pulse-like volume velocity functions at the neoglottis.

Reduction of amplitude levels in the 6000-9000 Hz region may be attributable to altered air pressure and flow associated with the generation of consonantal sounds due to limited power supply of the esophageal air reservoir and to oral compression mechanisms (Christensen and Weinberg 1976; Snidecor and Isshiki 1965). Further investigation of acoustic and aerodynamic characteristics of the neoglottis and altered vocal tract appears warranted.

It is clear that substantial differences were observed between the intensity and long-time spectral properties of esophageal and normal speech. The marked flattening of the long-time spectrum for esophageal speech, coupled with the relative flattening of the intensity distribution and the increased prevalence of lower intensity sound output associated with esophageal speech, is not unexpected. The production of esophageal speech is known to be associated with the production of less-periodic sound generation (Snidecor and Isshiki 1965; Smith et al. 1978).

The observed differences in the acoustic properties of esophageal and normal speakers suggest that additional attention might be devoted to evaluating the form of noise spectrum used in masking studies with esophageal speech. Finally, the differences in the spectral properties between these two very different forms of speech also serve to re-emphasize how radically the intensity of the speech spectrum may be altered without affecting its intelligibility.

Speech/Vocal Quality and Acceptability

There would be widespread agreement that esophageal speakers display a wide range of vocal quality characteristics. Despite this variability, all esophageal speakers have voices that have one common property, namely, the vocal quality of esophageal voice is not normal. This statement could be made for all types of alaryngeal speech. In view of the nature of the voicing sources used to support alaryngeal speech, normality should not be expected.

Weinberg and Bennett (1972) have provided information about the reasons listeners classify alaryngeal speakers as "non-normal." The principal reason cited is that the quality does not sound normal. Smith et al. (1978) have shown that the voices of esophageal speakers are rough, although the severity of perceived roughness varies from speaker to speaker. The factors underlying the production of rough-sounding vocal quality among these speakers is not well understood, although it is known that: (1) such voices are characterized by an increase in vocal jitter and shimmer; and (2) the voices of esophageal speakers are more noisy than normal. In addition to the rough and noisy quality, the voices of some esophageal speakers have a wet or bubbly quality; others are strained and tense.

Esophageal speakers may also produce a variety of extraneous sounds. The two most common sounds are (1) extraneous noises associated with air intake and (2) stomal noise. The presence of

Reasons Listeners Cited for Classifying Alaryngeal
Speakers as Nonnormal Speakers**

Esophageal Speech

Quality does not sound normal (53%)
Speech too slow (32%)
Pitch too low (24%)
Speech sounds mechanical (21%)
Voice is monotonous (19%)
Pitch is too high (3%)
Speech is too fast (3%)
Other: breathing sounds funny (1%)
    jagged, hesitant (3%)
    sounds harsh (1%)

Bell Electrolarynx Speech

Speech sounds mechanical (95%)
Quality does not sound normal (50%)
Voice is monotonous (47%)
Speech is too slow (28%)
Pitch is too low (11%)
Speech is too fast (6%)
Pitch is too high (3%)
Other: produced by machine (3%)
    robot (3%)

Western Electric Reed Speech

Quality does not sound normal (68%)
Speech is too slow (32%)
Speech sounds mechanical (31%)
Voice is monotonous (25%)
Pitch is too high (13%)
Pitch is too low (4%)
Speech is too fast (0%)
Other: nasal (3%)
    intoxicated (3%)

Tokyo Artificial Larynx Speech

Pitch is too low (48%)
Speech is too slow (41%)
Speech sounds mechanical (41%)
Voice is monotonous (27%)
Quality does not sound normal (20%)
Pitch is too high (4%)
Speech is too fast (0%)
Other: too dramatic (4%)

*Values reflect the percentage of listeners citing a given category to explain their response of "not a normal speaker."

such sounds detracts from the overall perceived acceptability of esophageal speech and signals deviancy or abnormalcy.

There is also the issue of identifying the determinants of overall acceptability of esophageal speech. The work of Shipp (1967) and Hoops and Noll (1969) has shown that variables such as speech rate, phonation time characteristics, and severity of stomal noise ratings are significantly related to judgments of speech acceptability. Taken together, this body of data reveals that the perceived, overall acceptability of esophageal speech increases as a function of decreasing the level of stomal noise, increasing speech rate, decreasing the amount of time speakers spend in silence, and increasing the amount of time speakers spend voicing. In a related vein, there is the issue of identifying factors that may limit or preclude either the acquisition of esophageal voicing or the development of functionally serviceable esophageal speech. This is not a trivial issue for clinical speech pathologists or surgeons. Shames, Font, and Matthews (1963) and others have sought to identify biographical, medical, personality-social, communication, and speech-training variables that correlated with speech proficiency. Comparative information about the relationship between these factors is also available for users of artificial larynges. Although significant relationships have been found between a sizable number of variables and speech proficiency, such data should not be interpreted to support the view that predictors for esophageal voice and speech acquisition have been established.

Comprehensive review of the literature on total laryngectomy and esophageal speech rehabilitation reflects a predominant interest in such areas as the diagnosis of laryngeal malignancy, surgical and nonsurgical treatment regimes, anatomical and physiological determinants of alaryngeal voice and speech production, and characteristics of speech after laryngectomy. Fundamental to any discussion of laryngeal malignancy, total laryngectomy, and speech rehabilitation is the fact that we are dealing with people. Hence, serious study of the topic of speech after laryngectomy must include an examination of such issues as patient's reactions to the diagnosis of laryngeal cancer and the subsequent surgery, presurgical and postoperative anxieties, fears, trauma and reactions to altered physical appearance, body state, related medical and social problems, and the extent to which psychosocial factors may relate to successful acquisition of speech after laryngectomy. For example, Duguay (1966) has provided useful information about the presurgical views of patients regarding the nature of their postsurgical speech. Duguay has highlighted some dramatic and, in some cases, pathetic, misconceptions harbored by patients and provided rehabilitation specialists with practical suggestions on alleviating those misconceptions. Gardner (1966) has discussed the special problems encountered by women undergoing total laryngectomy and alaryngeal speech rehabilitation. Amster et al. (1972) have provided a comprehensive examination of psychosocial factors and speech after laryngectomy. Their study, coupled with their extensive literature and bibliographic review, is essential reading for persons seriously interested in the problems of alaryngeal speech. More recently, Gilmore (1974) explored the social and vocational acceptability of esophageal speakers and normal speakers.

The results of these works reveal that esophageal speakers experience reductions in social and vocational status—an observation of considerable significance to all professionals involved in the treatment of laryngectomized patients.

Linguistic Aspects of Speech Following Total Laryngectomy

A major thesis developed in this chapter is that the effects of larynx removal are pervasive. It is, however, assumed that surgical removal of the larynx does not impair the linguistic form of the laryngeal speakers message. Namely, the syntactic, semantic, and phonological processes involved in the generation of utterances remain intact. On the other hand, it is assumed that all alaryngeal speakers employ altered strategies of speech production. Moreover, the extent to which "reprogramming" of the speech apparatus is possible in various abnormal speech-producing systems is expected to yield insight about the nature of intrinsic versus extrinsic properties of the acoustic signal and the psychological reality of abstract linguistic units and rules.

In this context, it is further assumed that all alaryngeal speakers have a nonconventional source of phonation; in addition, these speakers also have a nonconventional airstream mechanism. Hence, the extent to which alaryngeal speakers are able to realize various types of linguistic contrasts depends, in part, upon the specific properties upon which a given contrast is based and on the constraints of the altered speech-producing apparatus. For example, if a given distinction or contrast rests upon critical phonatory or airstream mechanisms, alaryngeal speakers must obviously reprogram the stages of signal generation that mediate this distinction. Variations in the ability to realize important types of linguistic contrasts are expected (1) between normal and alaryngeal speakers, and (2) among speakers using various types of alaryngeal speech. Hence, study of linguistic aspects of speech production by alaryngeal speakers is expected to provide insights into the nature of compensatory adjustments of the speech production apparatus that occur during the generation of contrastive speech patterns.

It is now evident that major types of linguistic contrasts are manifested in a complex form of acoustic and temporal cues. We assume that alaryngeal speakers reorganize the hierarchy of cues to conform to the physical constraints imposed by their altered speech-producing systems. In this regard, if the extrinsic manifestation of a given type of linguistic contrast depends upon some intrinsic property of the normal speech-producing system that is absent or altered in systems of alaryngeal speakers, one should be in a position to assess the nature of physical constraints that must be imposed upon alaryngeal models of speech production. At the same time, studies of linguistic aspects of speech after laryngectomy are expected to bring fresh data to bear on models of speech production/perception, in general.

It is apparent that the bulk of research and clinical study in alaryngeal speech has been descriptive in nature. Only recently have investigators been interested in examining, in a serious fashion, linguistic aspects of speech after laryngectomy. A review of some of this work should highlight the state of the art in this area of study and the important contributions that stem from studies of this type.

Productive VOT Characteristics

By way of example, it is now well known that normal speakers of English systematically vary the timing of voice onset to distinguish prevocalic stops /p, t, k/ from /b, d, g/ (Lisker and Abramson 1967). It is also now well established that laryngectomized patients using esophageal speech have difficulty achieving voicing contrast between homorganic stop consonants. These observations, coupled with the view that alterations in the speech-production systems of esophageal speakers create special problems in the control of temporal aspects of voicing, led Christensen, Weinberg and Alfonso (1978) to examine the variations in the timing of voice onset used by esophageal speakers. The distributions of measured voice onset times associated with the production of stops by esophageal and normal speakers are shown in Figures 1-9, 1-10, and 1-11. Examination of

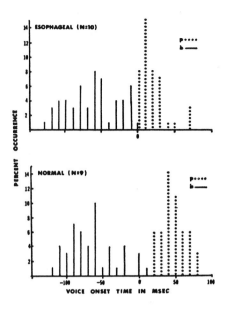

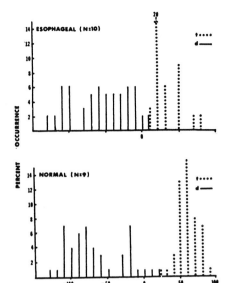

Figure 1-9.

Figure 1-10.

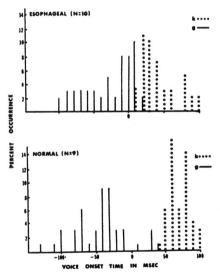

Figure 1-9. Distribution of voice onset times for labial stops.

Figure 1-10. Distribution of voice onset times for apical stops.

Figure 1-11. Distribution of voice onset times for velar stops.

Figure 1-11.

these data reveal that esophageal speakers did effect systematic variation in the timing of voice onset during the production of stops and that the VOT values associated with the production of prevocalic voiceless stops exhibited lag intervals that were significantly shorter than those used by normal speakers. These results also revealed that VOT characteristics of esophageal speakers were differentially sensitive to place of articulation.

Esophageal speakers systematically varied VOT during the production of phonetically representative speech sounds with the same manner of production, and the general pattern of these variations paralleled that observed for normal speakers. These findings were interpreted to support the belief that esophageal speakers employ variation within the voicing dimension to distinguish prevocalic stops /p, t, k/ from /b, d, g/.

Overlap was noted in the voice onset times associated with the production of homorganic stops, emphasizing that VOT represents one, but not the sole, acoustic property normal and esophageal speakers manipulate to distinguish effectively between homorganic stop consonants (Slis 1970; Slis and Cohen 1969*a*, *b*; Zlatin 1974, and others). Moreover, the observation of overlap, coupled with the disparity in absolute voice onset times between esophageal and normal speakers, particularly in prevocalic, voiceless stop productions, suggests that cues to voicing such as VOT should be regarded in a relative rather than an absolute manner.

The observation that esophageal speakers effected systematic variation in VOT is intriguing because of the striking differences between the voice- and speech-producing systems of normal and esophageal speakers. For example, it can be assumed that the phonatory aparatus of esophageal speakers does not possess abductor-adductor properties. The prevailing consensus is that differences within the voicing dimension reflect temporal aspects of glottal abductor-adductor activity operating in conjunction with articulatory and aerodynamic responses. Hence, it would be reasonable to expect that esophageal speakers might exhibit differences in VOT. Indeed, the earlier onset of esophageal voicing associated with voiceless stop production may reflect such changes and may highlight the

.1 contribution articulatory-aerodynamic responses
.n the timing of voicing onset. The earlier onset of
.ssociated with prevocalic voiceless stops also serves, in
.ccount for the lengthening of vowel duration observed for
this group of esophageal speakers (Christensen and Weinberg
1976).

These results were interpreted to support the view that
esophageal speakers are capable of effecting systematic and
linguisitically appropriate variation in the timing of voicing
onset. However, the extensive number of unrepresentative syllables uttered by esophageal speakers supports the hypothesis that
they are far less consistent than normal speakers in effecting
appropriate variation in the timing of voicing onset.

Vowel Duration Characteristics

One primary aim common to diverse studies of linguistic
aspects of speech after laryngectomy is to determine the degree to
which inherent, rule-governed features of English are retained
following laryngeal amputation. In this regard, it is well known
that vowel durations are conditioned by the voicing features of
their consonant contexts. Christensen and Weinberg measured
vowel durations from symmetric CVC syllables produced by ten
esophageal speakers. Some results of this work (*see* Figs. 1-12 and
1-13) revealed that the durations of vowels spoken by normal and
esophageal speakers in voiced consonant contexts were comparable. On the other hand, the durations of vowels spoken by
esophageal speakers within voiceless consonant contexts were
consistently longer than vowels spoken in similar contexts by
normal speakers. In addition, vowel durations spoken by esophageal speakers in voiced consonant contexts were always longer
than those uttered in voiceless consonant environments.

The results of this investigation indicate that total laryngectomy
also produces change in articulatory behavior, as evidenced by
altered durational characteristics of vowels. Moreover, that such
changes are influenced by phonetic context; namely, the observed
differences in vowel duration between normal and esophageal
speakers varied systematically as a function of the voicing
features of their consonant environment, and indicate that

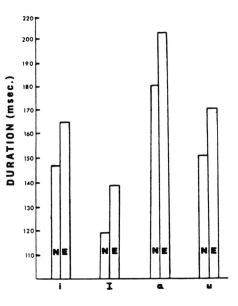

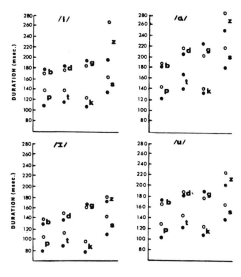

Figure 1-12. Comparison of overall mean vowel durations produced by esophageal (E) and normal (N) speakers.

Figure 1-13. Comparison of average durations of vowels produced by esophageal (open circles) and normal (closed circles) speakers. Values plotted as a function of consonant environment differences.

phonological rules governing the durational properties of English vowels are preserved following laryngeal amputation.

More recently, Gandour, Weinberg, and Rutkowski (1980) reexamined the influence of postvocalic consonants on vowel duration in esophageal speech. Due to the symmetrical nature of the stimuli and the measurement procedure used by Christensen and Weinberg, it is difficult to determine the real extent to which vowel length varied as a function of postvocalic consonant environment. Thus, here 18 C_1VC_f utterances were used. However, C_1 = /p/, V = /i, ɑ, u/, and C_f = /p, t, k, b, d, g/.

From a theoretical point of view, several competing hypotheses have been formulated to account for vowel-length variation. Some of these explanations involve adjustments of the larynx. Chomsky and Halle (1968) posit a vowel-lengthening rule before voiced stops, and Klatt (1976) gives a shortening rule before voiceless stops. Moreover, these investigators would say that these natural phonetic tendencies have apparently been expanded into a phonological rule of the grammar. In any event, if vowel-length variation induced by the voicing of the post-vocalic consonant environment in English is induced by inherent physiological characteristics of laryngeal (phonatory) adjustment, the prediction would be that this effect would not be present in esophageal speech. If, on the other hand, vowel-length variation is governed by a phonological rule in English, this effect should be evident, provided (1) that it is merely an expansion of some natural phonetic tendency of laryngeal (phonatory) adjustment and (2) the physiological control mechanisms underlying this effect are available to the esophageal speaker.

The results of our recent work again revealed that average durations of vowels were longer before voiced consonants than before voiceless consonants, for both esophageal and normal speakers. Thus, the influence of postvocalic consonants on vowel duration, previously observed in a population of normal speakers of American English (e.g. House and Fairbanks 1953; Peterson and Lehiste 1960; House 1961; Umeda 1975; Klatt 1976), is present in highly rated esophageal speakers. Not only is the effect of postvocalic consonants on vowel duration present in esophageal speech, but the magnitude of the effect is larger in esophageal speech when compared to normal speech.

House advanced the hypothesis that the lengthening of vowels before voiced consonants in English is a language-specific characteristic of the phonological system of the language. The differential influence of the consonant environment is not simply a function of inherent physiological features of the articulatory process, but is a language-specific speech characteristic learned by speakers of the language.

The results of this more recent investigation of vowel duration in esophageal speech provide additional support of the concept that these durational differences are learned by speakers of English. It is assumed that surgical removal of the larynx removes the normal source of phonation and substantially alters the means of speech production, but that the linguistic form of the speaker's message remains unimpaired. The finding that vowels before voiced consonants are longer than those before voiceless consonants in esophageal speech is expected only if it is assumed that these vowel-length variations are language-specific properties of the English phonological system. We would argue (1) that esophageal talkers "reprogram" neuromotor instructions required to implement this abstract phonological distinction in an abnormal speech-production system, and (2) that the extent to which such reprogramming is possible in conjunction with an altered speech apparatus clearly lends credence to the psychological reality of the abstract linguistic nature of the phenomenon.

Although absolute durations were greater for the esophageal group than for the normal group, relative increments in vowel duration in the environment of postvocalic consonants were not found to be significantly different. This finding lends further support for the abstract linguistic nature of the phenomenon. The esophageal talker apparently adopts a strategy of speech production that preserves this phonological distinction, despite the use of an alaryngeal speech apparatus. Only the speech apparatus, not the linguistic code, has been altered by laryngectomy. The esophageal talker presumably makes compensatory adjustments in the timing control system in order to realize these variations in vowel length before voiced and voiceless consonants.

In a broader perspective, these results show that data obtained from a clinically disordered population can be brought to bear on key notions associated with linguistic theory and models of speech production and perception.

Vowel Height and Fundamental Frequency

It has been established that the fundamental frequency (f_o) of vowels varies systematically as a function of vowel height (Crandall 1925; Black 1949; Peterson and Barney 1952; House and Fairbanks 1953; Lehiste and Peterson 1961; Ohala and Eukel 1971 for American English; Ladefoged 1968 for Itsekiri; Mohr 1971 for Chinese, German, and Russian; Gandour and Maddieson 1976 for Thai; Hombert 1977 for Yoruba; Petersen 1978 for Danish). Specifically, high vowels have a higher f_o than low vowels. Various explanations have been offered to account for this intrinsic variation in f_o between vowels. (For reviews of hypotheses see Atkinson 1973; Ohala 1973; Hombert 1978; Petersen 1978; Ewan 1979*a*, *b*).

Two major explanations or hypotheses dominate contemporary accounts offered to explain the mechanisms underlying intrinsic variation in vowel f_0. One of these is the source-tract coupling hypothesis (Lieberman 1970; Atkinson 1973). Proponents of this hypothesis account for the increase in f_0 for high vowels by postulating that when the frequency of the first formant of vowels is near the fundamental frequency of the source, acoustic coupling results between these vocal tract and source properties. In this situation, proponents argue that the lower frequency of the first formant attracts and raises the fundamental. Coupling does not occur when the frequency of the first formant is farther away from the voice fundamental frequency, as is the case for low vowels. Ohala (1973), Ewan (1979b), and others have offered evidence against this explanation.

The second explanation has been labeled the *tongue-pull hypothesis* (Ladefoged 1968; Lehiste 1970). Proponents of this argue that when the tongue is stretched or elevated to produce high vowels, a pull is exerted on the larynx altering the tension of the vocal folds, and consequently, an increase in f_0 results. The magnitude of transmission of tension from the tongue to the larynx is decreased during the production of low vowels. Although this explanation highlights anatomical interconnections between the tongue and the larynx, proponents of this hypothesis have encountered difficulty specifying the precise interconnections between the tongue and the larynx that mediate altered tension of the vocal folds. Lehiste (1970) suggested that the critical anatomical interconnection is the hyoid bone. Lindau, Jacobsen, and Ladefoged (1972) and Atkinson (1973) found that hyoid bone position is inversely related to vowel height. Such findings suggest that stretch or pulling may not be mediated through the hyoid bone, but leave open the possibility that pulling is mediated through other tissues.

Ohala (1973) suggested that pulling is accomplished via aryepiglottic tissues. Ohala and Eukel (1976) used a bite-block technique to test this version of the tongue-pull hypothesis. They found a small, but consistent increase in the difference in f_0

between high versus low vowels as a function of increasing jaw opening.

Ewan (1979*a, b*) has recently suggested a modification of the tongue-pull hypothesis which emphasizes compression of soft tissue above the vocal folds during the production of low vowels, rather than emphasizing pulling or stretching of the tongue during the production of high vowels. During the production of low vowels, Ewan argues that compression of the tongue and narrowing of the pharyngeal cavity results in an inferior displacement of tissue, which, in turn, brings about a slackening or decrease in vertical tension of the vocal folds, an increase in their effective vibrating mass, and a decrease in f_0.

It is clear that alternative and creative approaches are needed to isolate the mechanism(s) mediating intrinsic variations in vowel f_0. A project was undertaken to provide a novel approach to the study of this problem. In this experiment, data from esophageal speech produced by laryngectomized patients was used to provide a re-examination of the dominant contemporary hypotheses proposed to account for intrinsic vowel f_0 variation.

With surgical removal of the larynx, there is no question of hyoid influence mediating tongue pull on the tongue. Removal of the larynx necessitates removal of the hyoid and sacrifice of points of attachment of all suprahyoid and infrahyoid muscles. The voicing source used to support esophageal speech is the surgically altered pharyngoesophageal sphincter or segment, an aggregate structure we view as a surgical residue (Weinberg 1980).

We assume that there are no critical anatomical interconnections between the tongue and P-E segment that would systematically alter the properties of the P-E segment in relation to tongue height. The following anatomical and surgical information supports this assumption. The primary muscle of the P-E segment in normal man is the *cricopharyngeus*. In addition, muscular fibers of the upper esophagus (inner circular esophageal) and the lower pharynx (inferior constrictor muscle) also contribute to the formation of this sphincter (Zaino et al. 1970; Ellis 1971). Total laryngectomy surgery typically necessitates removal of all structures between the hyoid bone and the upper tracheal rings. Hence, the points of attachment of a large number of extrinsic laryngeal muscles, laryngeal membranes and ligaments, lower pharyngeal muscles, and the cricopharyngeus are sacrificed. Therefore, the assumption that no direct interconnection exists between the tongue and P-E segment that would mediate systematic variation in vowel f_o appears quite reasonable. If the tongue-pull hypothesis is correct, systematic differences in f_o between high versus low vowels produced by esophageal speakers would not be expected.

We also assume that the effects of acoustic coupling between the vocal tract and source are substantially, if not wholly, reduced in the circumstance of vowel production by esophageal speakers. For example, it is now well established that (1) the average f_o (65 Hz) of male esophageal voices is appreciably lower than that of the average nonlaryngectomized male, and (2) the formant frequencies of vowels produced by esophageal speakers are typically elevated in comparison with those produced by normal talkers (Weinberg and Bennett 1972; Sisty and Weinberg 1972). Hence, if the source-tract coupling hypothesis is correct, systematic differences in the f_o between high versus low vowels produced by esophageal speakers would also not be expected.

Four esophageal speakers provided recordings of fifteen tokens of three CVC syllables (hid, hud, had). The f_o and standard deviations (±1) values for each vowel produced by each speaker are illustrated in Figure 1-14. The absolute f_o of high vowels differed significantly from that for low vowels for three speakers. In the remaining speaker the difference failed to reach significance ($P = 0.056$).

The results of this study reveal that intrinsic variation in vowel f_o is clearly evident in esophageal speech. On either an absolute or relative basis, the magnitude of the differences in f_o between high and low vowels produced by esophageal speakers compared favorably with differences reported for normal speech. These results were interpreted to support neither the source-tract coupling nor the tongue-pull hypotheses. As indicated earlier, proponents of either of these theoretical positions would predict that the difference in f_o between high versus low vowels produced by esophageal speakers would be diminished.

Instead, the results of the present project indicate that the

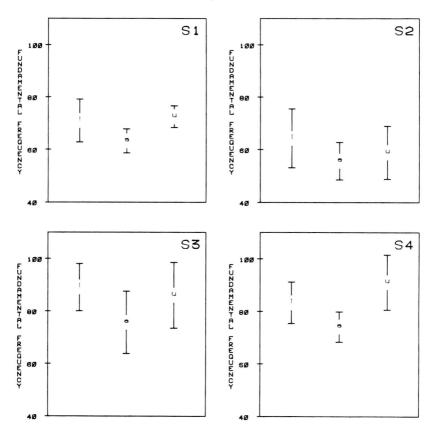

Figure 1-14. Fundamental frequency and standard deviation (1) values for vowels spoken by individual speakers S1-S4.

nature of intrinsic differences in f₀ between high and low vowels is substantially the same in esophageal and normal speech. Such results led us to offer an alternative explanation to account for these differences (Gandour and Weinberg 1980).

Briefly, we have speculated that the mechanism underlying the intrinsic variations in f₀ of vowels may be relatively simple. We have predicted that speakers exhibit a consistent increase in respiratory drive or speech effort during the production of high vowels versus low vowels. This increase merely reflects an involuntary adjustment or response to the slight elevation in vocal-tract impedance present during the production of high vowels.

Additional Forms of Linguistic Contrast

Synthesis of this review makes it apparent that systematic control of the frequency, durational, and intensity attributes of speech and voicing are critical to the realization of linguistic contrasts. Unfortunately, there is an absence of information concerning the ability of laryngectomized speakers to realize such important types of contrasts as stress, intonation, and juncture. We are currently engaged in a large-scale project to study fundamental aspects of stress, intonation, and juncture regulation among postlaryngectomy patients who use several forms of alaryngeal speech; unfortunately, only preliminary data are available. Thus, we have chosen not to explore this area, but to alert readers to this ongoing project. The major questions being addressed in this project include:

1. To what extent can alaryngeal speakers produce linguistically meaningful contrasts (stress, intonation, and juncture) in American English?
2. Are some alaryngeal speakers (esophageal, artificial larynx users, surgical-prosthetic speakers) more efficient in signalling given contrasts than others?
3. What are the specific acoustic and temporal parameters alaryngeal speakers use to signal contrasts?
4. Are these parameters comparable to those used by normal speakers?
5. Is there hierarchical ordering/reordering of cues used to signal contrasts?

The results of this project are expected to contribute critical information about the properties of speech that lead to successful/unsuccessful realization of important types of linguistic contrasts routinely used in speech. In addition, the results of this project are expected to lead us closer to the construction of models of alaryngeal speech or voice production and to the development of clinical procedures and materials designed to enhance prosody realization in alaryngeal speakers.

SUMMARY

In this chapter, a brief review of the mechanisms of alaryngeal speech and voice production has been provided. A detailed description of acoustical and temporal characteristics (fundamental frequency, intensity, long- and short-time spectra, rate, vocal quality, and extraneous sounds) of esophageal speech has been given together with a review of critical anatomical and physiological properties underlying esophageal speech/voice production. Finally, particular emphasis has been devoted to delineating linguistic aspects of speech after laryngectomy. Information has been interpreted to (1) provide insights about the precise nature of the impact occasioned by larynx removal in speech; (2) identify areas of information scarcity; and (3) highlight the role study of laryngectomized patients may play in solving important questions about speech production/perception in general.

REFERENCES

Amster, W.W., Love, R.J., Menzel, O.J., Sandler, J., Sculthorpe, W.B., and Gross, F.M.: Psychosocial factors and speech after laryngectomy. *J Commun Dis, 5*:1-18, 1972.

Angermeier, C., and Weinberg, B: Some aspects of fundamental frequency control by esophageal speakers. *J Speech Hear Res*, in press.

Atkinson, J.E.: Aspects of intonation in speech: Implications from an experimental study of fundamental frequency. Ph.D. diss., University of Connecticut (unpublished, 1973).

Barney, H.L.: A discussion of some technical aspects of speech aids for postlaryngectomized patients. *Ann Otol Rhinol Laryngol, 67*:558-570, 1958.

Barney, H.L., Haworth, F.E., and Dunn, H.K.: An experimental transistorized artificial larynx. *Bell System Tech J, 38*:1337-1356, 1959.

Bennett, S., and Weinberg, B.: Acceptability ratings of normal esophageal and artificial larynx speech. *J Speech Hear Res, 16*:608-615, 1973.

Black, J.W.: Natural frequency, duration and intensity of vowels in reading. *J Speech Hear Disorders, 14*, 216-221, 1949.

Calcaterra, T.C., and Jafek, B.W.: Tracheoesophageal shunt for speech rehabilitation after total laryngectomy. *Arch Otolaryngol, 94*:124-128, 1971.

Chomsky, N., and Halle, M.: *The Sound Pattern of English.* New York: MIT Pr 1968.

Christensen, J., and Weinberg, B.: Vowel duration characteristics of esophageal speech. *J Speech Hear Res, 19*:678-689, 1976.

Christensen J.M., Weinberg, B., and Alfonso, P.J.: Productive voice onset time characteristics of esophageal speech. *J Speech Hear Res, 21*:56-62, 1978.

Conley, J., DeAmesti, F., and Pierce, M.K.: A new surgical technique for the vocal rehabilitation of the laryngectomized patient. *Ann Otol Rhinol Laryngol, 67*:655-664, 1958.

Crandall, I.B., and MacKenzie, D.: Analysis of the energy distribution in speech. *Phys Rev, 19*: 221, 1922.

Crandall, J.B.:The sounds of speech. *Bell System Tech J, 4*:586-626, 1925.

Creech, H.B.: Evaluating esophageal speech, *J Speech Hear Assoc of Virginia, 7*: 13-19, 1966.

Curry, E.T., and Snidecor, J.C.: Physical measurement and pitch perception in esophageal speech. *Laryngoscope, 71*:415-424, 1961.

Curry, E.T., Snidecor, J.C., and Isshiki, N.: Fundamental frequency characteristics of Japanese asai speakers. *Laryngoscope, 83*:1759-1763, 1973.

Damste, P.H.: *Oesophageal Speech After Laryngectomy.* Groningen: Hoitsema, 1958.

Diedrich, W.: The mechanism of esophageal speech in sound production in man (A. Bouhuys, ed.). *Ann NY Acad Sci, 155*:303-317, 1968.

Diedrich, W.M., and Youngstrom, K.A.: *Alaryngeal Speech.* Springfield: Thomas, 1966.

Duguay, M.: Pre-operative ideas of speech after laryngectomy. *Arch Otolaryngol, 83*:69-72, 1966.

Dunn, H.F., and White, S.D.: Statistical measurements on conversational speech. *J Acoust Soc Am, 11*:278-288, 1940.

Ellis, F.J.: Upper-esophageal sphincter in health and disease. *Surg Clin North Am, 51*:553-565, 1971.

Ewan, W.G.: Laryngeal behavior in speech. *Rep Phonology Laboratory,* University of California, Berkeley, *3*: 1979a.

_____: Can intrinsic vowel F_0 be explained by source/tract coupling? *J Acoust Soc Am, 66*:358-362, 1979b.

Fredrickson, J.M., Charles, D.A., and Bryce, D.P.: An implantable electromagnetic sound source: Preliminary results of human implantation. Chapter 16 in *Surgical and Prosthetic Approaches to Speech Rehabilitation* (Shedd, D.P. and Weinberg, B., eds.) Boston: G.K. Hall, 1980.

Gandour, J., and Maddieson, I.: Measuring larynx movement in standard Thai using the cricothyrometer. *Phonetica, 33*:241-267, 1976.

Gandour, J., and Weinberg, B.: Influence of postvocalic consonants on vowel duration in esophageal speech. *Language and Speech, 23*:149-158, 1980.

_____: On the relationship between vowel height and fundamental frequency: evidence from esophageal speech. *Phonetica, 37*:344-354, 1980.

Gandour, J., Weinberg, B., and Rutkowski, D.: Influence of postvocalic consonants on vowel duration in esophageal speech. *Lang Speech, 23*: 149-158, 1980.

Gardner, W.H.: Adjustment problems of laryngectomized women. *Arch Oto-laryngol, 83:*31-42, 1966.

Gilmore, S.: Social and vocational acceptability of esophageal speakers compared to normal speakers. *J Speech Hear Res, 17:* 599-607, 1974.

Griffiths, C.M. and Love, J.T.: Neoglottic reconstruction after total laryngectomy. *Ann Otol Rhinol Laryngol, 87:*180-184, 1978.

Hombert, J.-M.: Consonant types, vowel height and tone in Yoruba. *Stud Afr Linguistics, 8:*173-190, 1977.

———: Consonant types, vowel quality and tone. In *Tone, A Linguistic Survey* (Fromkin, ed.) New York: Academic Press, 1978.

Hoops, H.R., and Noll, J.D.: Relationships of selected acoustic variables to judgments of speech proficiency. *J Commun Disord, 2:*1-13, 1969.

Horii, Y., House, A.S., Li, K.-P., and Ringel, R.L.: Acoustic characteristics of speech produced without oral sensation. *J Speech Hear Res, 16:*67-77, 1973.

Horii, Y., and Hughes, G.W.: Speech analysis by computer. *Proc Natl Electron Conf, 27:*74-79, 1972.

Horii, Y., and Weinberg, B.: Intelligibility characteristics of superior esophageal speech presented under various levels of masking noise. *J Speech Hear Res, 18:*413-419, 1975.

House, A.: On vowel duration in English. *J Acoust Soc Am, 33:* 1174-1178, 1961.

House, A., and Fairbanks, G.: The influence of consonant environment upon the secondary acoustical characteristics of vowels. *J Acoust Soc Am, 25:* 105-113, 1953.

Hyman, M.: An experimental study of artificial larynx and esophageal speech. *J Speech Hear Disord, 20:*291-299, 1955.

Isshiki, N., and Snidecor, J.C.: Air intake and usage in esophageal speech. *Acta Otolaryng, 59:*559-574, 1965.

Kirchner, J.A., Scatliff, J.H., Dey, F.L., and Shedd, D.P.: The pharynx after laryngectomy. *Laryngoscope, 73:*18-33, 1963.

Klatt, D.H.: Linguistic uses of segmental duration in English: Acoustic and perceptual evidence. *J Acoust Soc Am, 59:*1208-1221, 1976.

Komorn, R.M.: Vocal rehabilitation in the laryngectomized patient with a tracheo-esophageal shunt. *Ann Otol Rhinol Laryngol, 83:*445-451, 1974.

Kytta, J.: Spectrographic studies of the sound quality of esophageal speech. *Acta Otolaryng,* Suppl. 188, 1964.

Ladefoged, P.: *A Phonetic Study of West African Languages*; 2nd ed. New York: Cambridge University Press, 1968.

Lauder, E.: The laryngectomee and the artificial larynx. *J Speech Hear Dis, 33:* 147-157, 1968.

Lehiste, I.: Suprasegmentals. Cambridge, MA: MIT Press, 1970.

Lehiste, I., and Peterson, G.: Some basic considerations in the analysis of intonation. *J Acoust Soc Am, 33:*419-425, 1961.

Lieberman, P.: A study of prosodic features. *Haskins Lab Status Res Speech Res, 23:*179-208. New Haven: Haskins Laboratories, 1970.

Lindau, M., Jacobsen, L., and Ladefoged, P.: The feature advanced tongue root. *UCLA Working Papers in Phonetics, 22:*76-94, 1972.

Lisker, L., and Abramson, A.S.: Some effects of context on voice onset time in English stops. *Lang Speech, 10:*1-28, 1967.

McCroskey, R.L., and Mulligan, M.: The relative intelligibility of esophageal speech and artificial larynx speech. *J Speech Hear Dis, 28:*37-41, 1963.

Miller, A.H.: First experiences with the asai technique for vocal rehabilitation after total laryngectomy. *Ann Otol Rhinol Laryngol, 76:*829-833, 1967.

Mohr, B.: Intrinsic variations in the speech signal. *Phonetica, 23:*65-93, 1971.

Moolenaar-Bijl, A.: Connection between consonant articulation and intake of air in esophageal speech. *Folia Phoniatr, 5:*212-216, 1953.

Ohala, J.: Explanations for the intrinsic pitch of vowels. Monthly Internal Memorandum (January), Phonology Laboratory. Berkeley: University of California, 1973.

Ohala, J., and Eukel, B.W.: Explaining the intrinsic pitch of vowels. *Rep Phonology Laboratory* (Berkeley: University of California), *2:*118-125, 1978. [Abstract also in *J Acoust Soc Am, 60:*S44, 1976.]

Peterson, G., and Barney, H.L.: Control methods used in a study of the vowels. *J Acoust Soc Am, 24:*175-184, 1952.

Peterson, G., and Lehiste, I.: Duration of syllabic nuclei in English. *J Acoust Soc Am, 32:*693-703, 1960.

Petersen, N.R.: Intrinsic fundamental frequency of Danish vowels. *J Phonet, 6:*177-189, 1978.

Sacco, P.R., Mann, M.B., and Schultz, M.C.: Perceptual confusions among selected phonemes in esophageal speech. *J Ind Sp Hear Assoc, 26:*19-33, 1967.

Scarpino, J., and Weinberg, B.: Junctural contrasts in esophageal and normal speech. *J Speech Hear Res,* in press.

Shames, G.H., Font, J., and Matthews, J.: Factors related to speech proficiency of the laryngectomized. *J Speech Hear Disord, 28:*273-287, 1963.

Shedd, D.P., and Weinberg, B.: *Surgical-Prosthetic Approaches to Speech Rehabilitation.* Boston: G.K. Hall, 1980.

Shipp, T.: EMG of the pharyngoesophageal musculature during alaryngeal voice production. *J Speech Hear Res, 13:*184-192, 1970.

———: Frequency, duration and perceptual measures in relation to judgments of alaryngeal speech acceptability. *J Speech Hear Res, 10:*417-427, 1967.

Simpson, I.C., Smith, J.C.S., and Gordon, M.: Laryngectomy: the influence of muscle reconstruction on the mechanism of oesophageal voice production. *J Laryngol and Otol, 87:* 961-990, 1972.

Singer, M.I., and Blom, E.D.: An endoscopic technique for restoration of voice after laryngectomy. *Ann Otol Rhinol Laryngol, 89:*529-533, 1980.

Sisson, G.A., McConnel, F.M.S., Logemann, J.A., and Yeh, S.: Voice rehabilitation after laryngectomy. *Arch Otolaryngol, 101:*178-181, 1975.

Sisty, N., and Weinberg, B.: Formant frequency characteristics of esophageal speech. *J Speech Hear Res, 15*:439-448, 1972.

Slis, I.H.: Articulatory measurements on voiced, voiceless and nasal consonants. *Phonetica, 24*:193-210, 1970.

Slis, I.H., and Cohen, A.: On the complex regulating the voiced-voiceless destruction, II. *Lang Speech, 12*:80-102, 1969a.

————: On the complex regulating the voiced-voiceless destruction, I. *Lang Speech, 12*:141-155, 1969b.

Smith, B., Weinberg, B., Feth, L.L., and Horii, Y.: Vocal jitter and roughness characteristics of vowels produced by esophageal speakers. *J Speech Hear Res, 21*:240-249, 1978.

Snidecor, J.C. and Curry, E.T.: How effectively can the laryngectomee expect to speak? *Laryngoscope, 70*:62-67, 1960.

————: Temporal and pitch aspects of superior esophageal speech. *Ann Otol Rhinol Laryngol, 68*:1-14, 1959.

Snidecor, J.C., and Isshiki, N.: Air volume and air flow relationships of six male esophageal speakers. *J Speech Hear Dis, 30*:205-216, 1965.

Taub, S., and Bergner, L.H.: Air bypass voice prosthesis for vocal rehabilitation of laryngectomees. *Amer J Surg, 125*:748-756, 1973.

Tikofsky, R.S.: A comparison of the intelligibility of esophageal and normal speakers. *Folia Phoniatr, 17*:19-32, 1965.

Umeda, N.: Vowel duration in American English. *Journal of the Acoustical Society of America, 58*:434-445, 1975.

Vega, M.F.: Larynx reconstructive surgery—a study of three years' findings—a modified surgical technique. *Laryngoscope, 85*:866-881, 1975.

Weinberg, B.: *Readings in Speech Following Total Laryngectomy.* Baltimore: Univ Park, 1980.

Weinberg, B., and Bennett, S.: A study of talker sex recognition of esophageal voices. *J Speech Hear Res, 14*:391-395, 1971.

————: Selected acoustic characteristics of esophageal speech produced by female laryngectomees. *J Speech Hear Res, 15*:211-216, 1972.

Weinberg, B., and Bosma, J.F.: Similarities between glossopharyngeal breathing and injection methods of air intake for esophageal speech. *J Speech Hear Dis, 35*:25-32, 1970.

Weinberg, B., Horii, Y., and Smith, B.E.: Long time spectral and intensity characteristics of esophageal speech. *J Acoust Soc Am, 67*:1781-1784, 1979.

Weinberg, B., and Riekena, A.: Speech produced with the Tokyo artificial larynx. *J Speech Hear Disord, 38*:383-389, 1973.

Weinberg, B., Shedd, D., and Horii, Y.: Reed-fistula speech following pharyngolaryngectomy. *J Speech Hear Res, 43*:401-413, 1978.

Winans, C.S., Reichbach, E.J., and Waldrop, W.G.: Esophageal determinants of alaryngeal speech. *Arch Otolaryngol, 99*:10-14, 1974.

Young, K.A., Bailey, B.J., Everett, R., and Griffiths, C.M.: Electronic laryngeal prosthesis for implantation: A progress report. Chapter 15 in *Surgical and Prosthetic Approaches to Speech Rehabilitation* (Shedd, D.P., and Weinberg, B., eds.) Boston: G.K. Hall, 1980.

Zaino, C., Jacobson, H.G., Lepow, H., and Ozturk, G.H.: *The Pharyngo-Esophageal Sphincter.* Springfield: Thomas, 1970.

Zlatin, M.A.: Voicing contrast: Perceptual and productive voice onset time characteristics of adults. *J Acoust Soc Am,* 59:981-994, 1974.

Chapter 2

COMPUTER ANALYSIS
OF ALARYNGEAL SPEECH

Yoshiyuki Horii

ABSTRACT

This chapter reviews some acoustic variables investigated for early detection of laryngeal pathologies and discusses computer methods of aerodynamic/acoustic analyses of alaryngeal speech developed by this author. Preliminary results of acoustic analysis are presented by using voice samples selected from a commercially available phonograph of alaryngeal speech. Problems of automatic acoustic analysis of alaryngeal speech are also discussed.

INTRODUCTION

F OR MANY YEARS, acoustic analysis has contributed to the understanding of production, transmission, and perception of normal and disordered speech. In more recent years, a number of mathematical techniques of speech analysis using computers have been developed and utilized to extract sound source and resonance characteristics of speech (Gold 1962; Atal and Schroeder 1968; Henke 1969; Denes 1970; Oppenheim 1970; Mermelstein 1971; Schafer 1970; Wakita 1972). These include the cepstrum method, co-variance and autocorrelation methods, the PARCOR method, the linear-prediction method, and the inverse filtering method, to name a few (Noll 1964; Itakura and Saito 1968; Atal and Hanauer 1971; Makhoul and Wolf 1972, Markel

---

This chapter was supported in part by the National Institute on Aging, Grant No. R01 AG01590.

and Gray 1973). In one way or another, these methods permit researchers to extract from the time-domain speech waveform, voice fundamental frequency (fo), harmonic amplitudes, formant frequencies, intensity, and the long-time and short-time spectrum of connected speech. High fidelity of these analysis methods has been demonstrated not only by the close agreements of their results with traditional spectrographic and oscillographic results, but also by highly intelligible synthesis results.

In spite of their potential as a diagnostic and evaluative tool, the computer methods have not been applied extensively to analysis of alaryngeal speech; that is, acoustic analysis of alaryngeal speech has been most frequently conducted using traditional spectrographic and oscillographic methods. One reason for this appears to be researchers' familiarity with these traditional methods over the mathematical and computerized methods of analysis. Another reason is that often those who developed the mathematical or computer methods were more interested in conceptual, theoretical aspects of the new methodology than in its practical applications and considerations geared toward "naive" users. In this respect, recent availability of user-oriented acoustic analysis systems (such as the ILS package by Signal Technology, Inc.*) is a welcome trend. Another reason, related to this and possibly more important, appears to be the difficulties of analyzing alaryngeal speech because of its divergent and deviant acoustic characteristics. Most computer techniques, developed and tested using normal speech, often require modifications to handle specific acoustic parameters of interest unique to alaryngeal speech analysis.

What appears to be urgently needed, then, is the exchange of information between those who work on software for general speech analysis and those who deal with alaryngeal speech. Mutual interest and effort should help to fill the gap between the theory and practice of computer-assisted analysis of alaryngeal speech. The purpose of this chapter, as suggested by the title, is to review methods and results of computer analysis of alaryngeal speech. Review of the literature, however, revealed few studies in

---

*15 W. De la Guerra Street, Santa Barbara, California, 93101.

this area. Thus, the review was expanded to include a brief discussion of computer-assisted acoustical analysis for early detection of laryngeal pathologies. Problems of acoustic analysis of alaryngeal speech by computer methods are also considered, using voice samples selected from a commercially available phonographic record.

EARLY DETECTION OF LARYNGEAL PATHOLOGY BY ACOUSTIC ANALYSIS

One physical aspect that has been considered to be sensitive enough to reflect laryngeal pathology in its early stage of development is aperiodicity of vocal-fold vibration. In contrast to healthy vocal folds, pathologic folds with benign or malignant tumors, for example, tend to produce less-periodic vibration. This has been observed in high-speed laryngoscopic motion pictures, as well as in acoustic signals (Scripture 1906; Simon 1927; Moore and Von Leden 1958; Von Leden, Moore and Timake 1960; Zemlin 1962; Moore and Thompson 1965; Jacob 1968; Beckett 1969; Hollien, Michel and Doherty 1973; Kitajima 1973; Smith 1976; Hiki et al. 1976). Thus, attempts have been made to measure the degree of periodicity during speech from acoustic signals.

The periodicity measures may be grouped into two general types: measures of voice f_o variations and measures of amplitude variations. These may be further subdivided into (1) variations around mean f_o or amplitude, and (2) cycle-to-cycle f_o (jitter) or amplitude (shimmer) variations. In addition to these independent f_o or amplitude measures, some attempts have been made to examine noise components in the voice through spectral analysis (Isshiki, Yanagihara, and Morimoto 1966; Yanagihara 1967a; Yanagihara 1967b; Iwata and Von Leden 1970; Emanuel, Lively and McCoy 1973; Deal and Emanuel 1978), or through residue analysis of inverse filtering (Koike and Markel 1975; Davis 1976) where both f_o and amplitude variations are presumably taken into account simultaneously.

There have been a large number of studies that examined vocal periodicity characteristics of normal and disordered speech using oscillographic, spectrographic, and/or photographic methods. However, only a limited number of studies exist where acoustical analysis methods were employed for early detection of laryngeal pathologies. The work by Lieberman and his colleagues (Lieberman 1961; Lieberman and Michaels 1962; Lieberman 1963; Smith and Lieberman 1969) was probably one of the first to attempt detection of laryngeal pathologies by waveform analysis. In essence, Lieberman examined cycle-to-cycle differences of periods in successive vocal-fold vibrations using continuous photographs of acoustic waveforms displayed on an oscilloscope. Measurements of periods and calculations of period differences were conducted by a digital data reduction system. The procedures involved visual inspection of the waveform and manual setting of a fine vernier to demarcate individual periods. The vernier setting was then transferred to computer cards through the reduction system. Lieberman reported a temporal resolution of 0.05 msec for this analysis method.

Through the analysis of connected speech produced by normal and pathological subjects (with laryngeal polyps, nodules, and cancer), Lieberman suggested a "perturbation factor" as an indicator of laryngeal pathologies. The perturbation factor was defined as the percentage of times the cycle-to-cycle differences were equal to or greater than 0.5 msec. Because the mean fo varies greatly among individuals, especially between males and females and between adults and children, the perturbation factor with such a fixed size of period difference turned out to be not very fruitful. After detailed oscillographic analysis of five patients, Hecker and Kreul (1971) suggested use of a "directional perturbation factor" as another index of laryngeal pathology. The directional perturbation factor was defined as the percentage of times the arithmetic sign of cycle-to-cycle period differences changed during speech. Hecker and Kreul reported greater occurrences of sign changes among the patients with laryngeal pathology. In addition, they suggested use of other measures such as fo standard deviation, phonation time ratio, and rate of utterances to discriminate normal and pathological voices.

Probably one of the most extensive periodicity studies of pathological voices was conducted by Crystal et al. (1970). They derived a total of 40 vocal quality indices (including the cycle-to-cycle period and amplitude differences) from connected speech and sustained /ɑ/ produced by 172 normal and 52 pathological larynges. The heart of their approach was a running prediction of pitch-peak amplitude and position and computation of the error between the predicted and the actual values. They have examined, for example, not only the period or amplitude differences of adjacent cycles, but also every other cycle or several consecutive cycles. They reported a reasonable success in discriminating normal and pathological larynges, especially for men using these indices.

Both the work by Lieberman and by Hecker and Kreul dealt with connected speech. Interpretation of the f_o analysis results is complicated in such speech materials, because both systematic f_o changes due to intonation, stress, phonetic contexts, etc., and rather random variations due to irregular vibratory characteristics caused by physical-structural properties of vibrating source co-exist. Although a possibility of enhanced manifestation of laryngeal aperiodicity when coupled to dynamic vocal-tract movements cannot be denied, many researchers concentrated their efforts on investigation of sustained vowel phonations.

Using sustained /ɑ/ phonations produced by patients with laryngeal tumors and paralysis, Koike (1973) examined average cycle-to-cycle differences of periods. The period measurements were made from oscillographic tracings of the voice signals picked up by a contact microphone placed between the thyroid and sternal notch. Noting slow modulations of f_o in many voices, Koike employed period deviations from the average of three cycles instead of deviations from preceding cycles. He reported average perturbations of 0.1 to 0.8 percent for normal subjects, 0.4 to 6.0 percent for tumor cases, and 0.5 to 3.5 percent for the paralysis cases in the midsegments of the phonations. He also reported much greater perturbation at the initial segments of phonation as might be expected.

Cycle-to-cycle amplitude variations, often called "shimmer," is another variable that reflects the less-periodic nature of pathologic larynges. Studies by Kitajima and Gould (1976) and by Koike (1969) may be cited as examples of the effort to detect laryngeal pathology from shimmer analysis. Kitajima and Gould examined average shimmer of 45 normal males and females and 25 with laryngeal polyps of different sizes and locations as they sustained vowel /ɑ/. The voice signals were low-passed at 1500 Hz and quantized at a rate of 20,000 times per second using a 10-bit, analog-to-digital converter. Due to limited core size, each sampled voice was 360 msec in duration. Measurements were made from oscillographic displays of the quantized data and by use of a cursor that was positioned manually. The cursor positions were stored and used for period calculations. In order to reduce slow modulations of amplitude, actual amplitude values used for calculation of shimmer were adjusted employing a least square linear fit to the five data points. (As discussed earlier, such an approach to reduce effects of slow modulations by a sort of moving average filter was also used by Koike (1973) and in a way by Crystal et al. (1970).) A system noise floor of up to about 0.1 db was reported for this analysis method. Their results showed that normal subjects had an average shimmer of 0.04 to 0.21 db with a critical value (0.05 level) of 0.19 db. Vocal shimmer in 25 subjects with polyps ranged from 0.08 to 3.23 db, with small overlap with the distribution of shimmer values for the normals.

A slightly different approach was also taken by Koike (1973) and Von Leden and Koike (1970) who employed a correlational analysis of time series data and examined amplitude modulations depicted in the resulting correlograms. In this approach, the oscillographic measurements of pitch-peak amplitudes were made from the most stable portion of sustained /ɑ/ phonations. Peak amplitudes for at least thirty consecutive cycles were used for correlational analysis for each lag between one and fifteen fundamental periods. Resulting series of correlation coefficients were called *correlograms*, which showed the serial correlation coefficient as the *ordinate* and the fundamental periods as the *abscissa*. Results showed that high correlations were often found between the consecutive dominant amplitude peaks and that the correlograms for patients with laryngeal neoplasms often displayed strong periodicities of amplitude modulations with periods of three to twelve fundamental periods. The paralysis cases, on the other hand, showed no evidence of periodic modulations in the same range.

Finally, an approach using inverse filtering techniques may be mentioned. Davis (1976) and Koike and Markel (1975) employed :he residue analysis of glottal waves derived by mathematically subtracting vocal-tract resonances from the acoustic waves recorded in front of the mouth. It may be said, however, that in general, the quantitative representation of the index for the level of noisiness in the residue signal or periodicity is yet to be investigated. Similarly, there are other acoustic aspects that appear to be quite relevant in analysis of laryngeal pathologies, such as spectral noise levels or inharmonic noise levels (Isshiki, Yanagihara, and Morimoto 1966; Yanagihara 1967a; Yanagihara 1967b; Iwata and Von Leden 1970; Emanuel, Lively, and McCoy 1973; Deal and Emanuel 1978). To the author's knowledge, computer extractions of such measures are also yet to be developed.

In lieu of a summary of this section, it should be emphasized that the purpose of the analysis largely dictates the specific acoustic parameters to be investigated. As seen in the studies reviewed above, primary concern in early detection of laryngeal pathologies has been directed toward analysis of laryngeal sound source characteristics rather than resonance characteristics of the vocal tract. In addition, although the computer has been employed at one stage or another of the analysis methods, completely automatic methods are as yet unavailable. To this end, the present author has developed a peak-picking f_0 analysis program called *SEARP*. Normative data for jitter, shimmer, and directional perturbation factors of jitter and shimmer, in addition to various f_0 distribution statistics, have just begun to accumulate (Horii 1975; Horii 1979; Horii 1980; Wilcox and Horii 1980; Sorensen and Horii, in press; Ramig, Ringel, and Horii, in press). The program will be described later as it was used to generate preliminary acoustic analysis results for alaryngeal speech.

AERODYNAMIC ANALYSIS OF
ALARYNGEAL SPEECH BY COMPUTER

Removal of the larynx not only produces a lack of the usual means of phonation, but also brings about changes in the airstream mechanisms required for the sound generation. Thus, investigation of aerodynamic aspects of alaryngeal speech plays an important role in the evaluation of a new speech-production method employed by the laryngectomized individuals, be it an intrinsic or a prosthetic method. The following is a description of the computer-assisted airflow, volume, and pressure analysis method developed by this author (Horii and Cooke 1978).

Figure 2-1 shows a block diagram illustrating the aerodynamic data collection procedures. Part A in the figure shows the signal recording procedure, while Part B illustrates the digitization procedure. As shown in Part A, oronasal airflow is funneled through a face mask to a pneumotachometer. Pressure differences across the mesh screen in the pneumotachometer are sensed and amplified by a bridge amplifier-pressure transducer system and recorded on one channel of a multi-channel FM tape recorder. Intraoral pressure or pressure inside an extrinsic pneumatic-type artificial larynx is sensed by a catheter and recorded on another channel of the recorder. Finally, voice signals are recorded on the third channel.

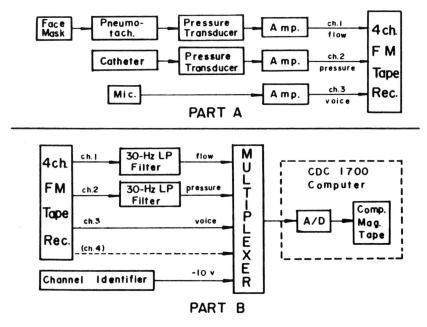

Figure 2-1. A block diagram illustrating the aerodynamic data collection procedures: (A) signal recording; (B) digitization.

Both flow and pressure signals are low-pass filtered at 30 Hz before digitization (Part B). The purpose of the low-pass filtering is to reduce voice fundamental frequency components. In addition to flow, pressure, and voice, one extra channel (currently empty) and channel identifier of –10V DC are also digitized by a 16-bit, analog-to-digital converter at 5,000 times per second, resulting in a 1 kHz sampling rate for each channel. The digitized data are continuously written on computer magnetic tape through a chaining buffer.

A program called *RESPAN* operates on the digitized airflow data. The volume velocity function during speech typically consists of large negative portions corresponding to inhalation and slowly varying positive DC signals (phonetic and syllabic components) superimposed by higher-frequency AC components (voice fundamental frequency for voiced segments). Specific functions of the program were (1) to detect inhalation and exhalation, (2) to calculate total inhaled and exhaled air volume for each breath group, (3) to obtain the time ratio of contiguous inhalation and exhalation, (4) to generate piecewise linear approximation of the volume velocity function, and (5) to calculate the maximum, minimum, and average rate of air usage for closure-to-closure segments (segments between a point of zero volume velocity to the next zero volume velocity during speech) within each breath group.

The program performs as a combination of peak, valley, plateau detector, zero detector, and inhalation detector. Primary programming consideration was given to reject the high-frequency (voice fundamental frequency and quantization noise) components in a peak-valley-plateau detection and to process multi-channel signals of virtually unlimited length. The multi-channel processing has been implemented into the program because of frequent needs to simultaneously investigate airflow, air volume, and voice signals. In addition, the program accomplishes derivation of all the measurements conventionally obtained by visual inspection and hand measurements of oscillographic records of airflow and volume signals during speech. Statistical data (histograms and the mean and standard deviation of instantaneous volume velocity) are also printed out at the end of the analysis. Optionally, the volume velocity function, its piecewise approximation, and the speech waveform can be displayed on an oscilloscope or on a multi-channel graphic-level recorder.

Using this procedure, Weinberg, Shedd, and Horii (1978) reported some airflow and volume data of reed-fistula and artificial larynx (Servox®) speakers. Figure 2-2 shows oscillograms of oronasal airflow and voice signals derived from normal subjects (top) and two reed-fistula subjects (center and bottom) during connected utterances. The different nature of oronasal flow between normal and reed-fistula speakers becomes evident. The reed-fistula speakers showed more frequent abrupt, high airflow rates, and obviously, no clear inhalatory events.

Figure 2-3 illustrates oronasal airflow and voice signals of a patient using an electrolarynx (Servox). Airflow is characterized by both negative and positive small flow that reflects volume changes of oral/pharyngeal cavities during speech. Again, no inhalatory events are visible as expected.

Results of airflow analysis associated with sustained phonation of a vowel /ɑ/ are shown in Table 2-I. Two reed-fistula subjects were asked to sustain phonation of /ɑ/ under three different conditions: (1) at a comfortable level of intensity, (2) at the lowest effort level necessary to activate and maintain sustained vibration of the reed mechanism, and (3) at the highest possible effort level permissible to maintain sustained voicing.

Table 2-I. Mean Airflow Rates (cc/sec) Associated with
Prolonged Phonation of a Vowel /ɑ/

	RF #1	RF #2	Normal	Esophageal*
At a Comfortable Intensity Level	211	196	150	27-72
Lowest Flow Rate	106	147	40	
Highest Flow Rate	251	248	250**	

*Isshiki and Snidecor, 1964.
**Produced with considerably higher intensity levels than the RF phonations.

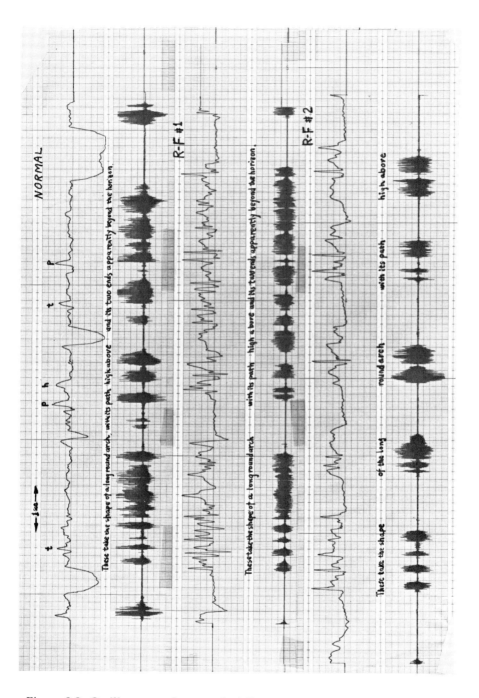

Figure 2-2. Oscillograms of oronasal airflow and voice signals derived from a normal (top) and two reed-fistula subjects (center and bottom) during connected utterances.

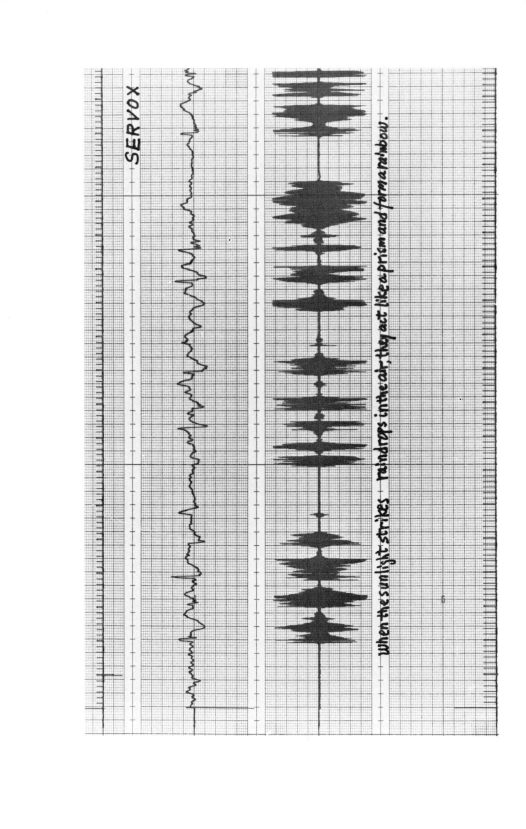

SERVOX

When the sunlight strikes raindrops in the air, they act like a prism and form a rainbow.

The data in Table 2-I indicate that at comfortable levels of speech intensity or effort, average airflow rate was about 200 cc/sec. On the other hand, flow rates associated with minimal activation and sustained voicing were about 100 cc/sec for Subject 1 and about 150 cc/sec for Subject 2. Flow rate associated with maximal effort and sustained voicing was about 250 cc/sec. These observations suggest that reed-fistula talkers are, from an aerodynamic point of view, rather limited to the higher end of the airflow continuum. For example, normal talkers sustain voicing with airflow rate as low as about 50 cc/sec at low intensity and use about 150 cc/sec airflow at a comfortable level of intensity (Isshiki 1964). At relatively high intensity, normal talkers typically use about 250 cc/sec airflow, although rates as high as 350 cc/sec have been reported for extremely high-intensity phonations (Isshiki 1964; Shipp and McGlone 1971). Snidecor and Isshiki (1965) reported airflow rates of 27 to 72 cc/sec during prolonged esophageal phonation of /ɑ/ at comfortable levels of production.

Airflow and volume characteristics associated with the oral reading of a standard passage are summarized in Table 2-II. For comparative purposes, data for a normal male and esophageal talkers are also provided. Reed-fistula speakers were clearly characterized by higher mean airflow rates and, consequently, higher total and syllabic volume air consumption. As expected, comparable aerodynamic characteristics for esophageal talkers are considerably smaller than observed for normal and reed-fistula talkers.

The distributional properties of sampled airflow rates associated with paragraph reading are shown in Figure 2-4. In this figure, the relative number of occurrences is plotted against the airflow rates in cc/sec to form a *frequency distribution curve*. Comparable data obtained from a normal male talker are also shown. Since one of the talkers (Speaker 2) was also an effective electrolarynx user, airflow distributional properties measured for speech produced with an artificial larynx (Servox) are also plotted. Clearly, reed-fistula talkers also used high airflow rates

←——

Figure 2-3. Oscillograms of oronasal airflow and voice signals of a patient using an electrolarynx (Servox).

Table 2-II. Airflow and Volume Characteristics Associated
with Oral Reading of a Passage

	RF #1 (M)	Normal (M)	RF #2 (F)	Normal (F)	Esophageal*
Maximum Volume Available	VC	VC	VC	VC	50-150 cc
Mean Airflow Rate	266 cc/sec	187 cc/sec	197 cc/sec	152 cc/sec	25-100 cc/sec
Total Volume Out	8154 cc	5351 cc	9360 cc	--	871-1115 cc
Total Speaking Time	44 sec	35 sec	75 sec	--	--
Volume/syllable	67 cc/syll	43 cc/syll	76 cc/syll	--	5-16 cc/syll

*Isshiki and Snidecor, 1964, 1965.

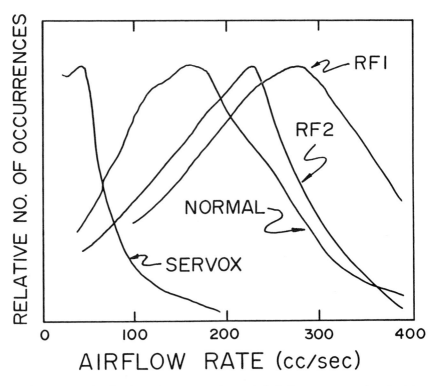

Figure 2-4. Distribution histograms of sampled airflow rates associated with paragraph reading.

in oral reading. Normal talkers would have to speak at production levels three times greater than normal to produce airflow distributions comparable to reed-fistula talkers. The airflow distributions of normal and reed-fistula speakers are comparable when normal talkers read the passage in a whisper (Cooke and Horii 1975). These observations emphasize the contributions aerodynamic studies may make to the design and evaluation of prosthetic speech devices.

ACOUSTIC ANALYSIS OF ALARYNGEAL SPEECH BY COMPUTER

In this section, preliminary results of alaryngeal speech analysis by a computer method are described. The computer program, SEARP, was developed by this author primarily for the f_o analysis of sustained phonations and connected speech produced by normal speakers (Horii 1975; Horii and Hughes 1972). The program was employed here without any modifications specific to alaryngeal speech analysis.

The program uses a peak-picking method and periodicity criteria in identifying voicing, unvoicing, and pause and, if voiced, its fundamental frequency from the time-sampled acoustic waveform. Voice signals recorded through a regular or contact microphone were quantized via a 16-bit, analog-to-digital converter at a nominal rate of 10,000 times per second (20,000 or 40,000 times per second for jitter analysis) and written continuously onto computer magnetic tape using a chaining buffer.

Program SEARP subsequently analyzes the digitized speech. Its output includes (1) a "melody plot" (optional), (2) total speaking time, (3) pause time, (4) the phonation time ratio, (5) f_o histogram and its descriptive statistics, (6) the perturbation function, (7) a jitter histogram and its descriptive statistics, including the directional perturbation factor, and (8) a shimmer and directional shimmer factor. The descriptive statistics derived from the f_o histogram include the mean, median, and mode, standard deviation, mid-90 percent range, mid-50 percent range, and total range. Most of these parameters are calculated both in Hz and in semitones. Reliability and validity of this method has been repeatedly tested and found satisfactory through analyses of various normal and disordered speech (Horii 1975; Horii 1979; Horii 1980; Wilcox and Horii 1980; Sorensen and Horii in press; Ramig, Ringel, and Horii in press; Zlatin-Laufer and Horii 1977; Weinberg, Dexter, and Horii 1975).

As stated earlier, the preliminary results reported here mainly came from a phonographic record entitled "Speech After Removal of the Larynx," by Dr. Harm A. Drost of the Phonetic Laboratory of the Ear, Nose, and Throat Department of the University Hospital, Leiden, the Netherlands.* The commercially available record was used in a hope that results of various analysis systems developed at different laboratories could be compared and evaluated on the same voice samples.

A summary of automatic analysis results for selected voice samples from the phonograph is presented in Table 2-III. In this table, mean f_o, f_o standard deviation, mid-90 percent range, total speaking time, percent of pause time, and percent of periodicity detected are shown for normal (Dr. Drost), parabuccal, esophageal, Pipa di Tichioni (artificial larynx), and Western Electric artificial larynx speech. Duration of sampled speech was arbitrarily determined and indicated by the total speaking time.

Table 2-III. A Summary of the Automatic Analysis Results for Selected Voice Samples of the Phonograph.

	Normal	Parabuccal	Esophageal	Pipa	Western Electric
Mean f_o (Hz)	148.9	188.1	86.5	61.0	81.2
f_o standard deviation (semitone)	4.25	2.18	3.29	0.64	0.24
Mid-90% range (semitone)	13.32	6.83	11.34	1.61	0.41
Total speaking time (sec)	27.0	37.4	30.6	55.4	32.4
Pause time (%)	34.0	(0)	38.3	37.2	(0)
% Periodic	64.3	49.7	64.2	75.5	97.2

*The record was distributed through Folkways Records and Service Corporation in New York.

Although not listed, rate of utterance in words per minute or syllables per minute could be easily calculated knowing the specific utterances.

It might be mentioned that Dr. Drost narrated with such an extremely well-modulated intonation that semitone values for f_0 standard deviation and mid-90 percent range were almost twice as large as those typically reported for adults' oral reading (Horii 1975; Mysak 1959; Bowler 1964). Spectrographic examination of his speech showed in fact that Dr. Drost often used more than one octave range in his utterances.

Parabuccal speech had a relatively high mean f_0 and very low percent periodicity values. The low percent periodicity was probably due to zero pause time that resulted from the high background noise (more specifically, poor speech-to-noise amplitude ratio). Esophageal speech, on the other hand, produced comparable values to the normal speech on all measures except its low mean f_0. (Rate of utterance and intensity levels, which were not shown in the table, were also clearly lower for esophageal speech than for normal speech.)

Rather limited f_0 variability was evident in the two examples of artificial larynx speech. Percent periodicity detected was high in these speech samples, particularly for the Western Electric artificial larynx speaker. The vibrator was on throughout his speech, resulting in zero pause time and practically 100 percent periodicity.

As stated earlier, these results are preliminary because no "tune-up" of the program was made for the types and recording conditions of these alaryngeal speech samples, and because detailed comparisons of these computer results and oscillographic hand measurements are yet to be made. Insight into possible problems of automatic computer analysis of alaryngeal speech may be gained, however, by examining spectrographic and oscillographic displays of these voices. Several comments on computer analysis of alaryngeal speech, therefore, may be made with the aid of wide-band and narrow-band spectrograms and digital oscillograms.

First, as with any type of speech analysis, good signal-to-noise ratio is of primary importance. Unfortunately, most alaryngeal speakers tend to have unfavorable signal-to-noise ratio because of (1) typically lower speech intensities, and (2) frequent introduction of extraneous noise (such as stoma noise and air injection noise). Thus, proper positioning of the microphone and optimal use of dynamic range of the recording and analysis equipment become important considerations. In addition, if stoma noise is relatively high, or sound leak at the skin contact of the electromechanical artificial larynx is prominent, for example, a compromise adjustment of the silence threshold has to be made in the automatic analysis program. Segments of the Western Electric speech and the parabuccal speech are shown in Figures 2-5 and 2-6 as an example. Because of considerable sound leak and poor signal-to-noise conditions, pause was not detected with the usual silence threshold. Pause time and phonation time ratio are particularly vulnerable to the poor signal-to-noise ratio and adjustment of the silence threshold.

Second, many intrinsic forms of alaryngeal speech such as buccal, parabuccal, and esophageal speech are often characterized by less-periodic vibrations of the neoglottis, even during sustained vowel phonations. Oftentimes, visual inspection of oscillographic displays of these voices fails to detect periodicity in the signals. Spectrographic and oscillographic displays for the glossopharyngeal and esophageal speech are shown in Figures 2-7 and 2-8.

Another point to consider is divergent f_0 characteristics of alaryngeal speech. Typically, average f_0 of esophageal speech is about 60 Hz. (Another reason to have good recording conditions so that line frequency or 60 Hz hum does not contaminate analysis results.) Parabuccal speech shown in Figure 2-9, on the other hand, has an average f_0 of about 350 Hz. Thus, analysis programs have to be able to handle a wide range of f_0 or at least be able to tune-in to different frequency regions. (Program SEARP currently has the capability to handle f_0 from 1 Hz to 600 Hz.) Many extrinsic forms of artificial larynges, fortunately from an analysis point of view, have highly periodic sources. Examples of larynxo-phone and Pipa di Tichioni speech are shown in Figures 2-10 and 2-11. Users of such devices, however, often face difficulties in voicing-unvoicing distinctions, especially for voiceless fricative productions.

The preliminary results reported above were made from speech signals low-passed at approximately 5000 Hz. One consideration would be to preprocess the signal by much more severe low-pass, such as 100 Hz or 200 Hz low-pass filtering. Such severe low-pass filtering would make algorithms of f_0 tracking simpler and possibly more accurate in periodicity detection. Another alternative is to use a contact microphone or miniature accelerometer as suggested by Koike (1973) and Stevens et al. (1975). The contact microphone in such applications serves two purposes: (1) low-pass filtering and (2) attenuation of extraneous noise. Preliminary investigations indicated that f_0 analysis results of voice recordings made by a contact microphone (BBN Piezoelectric Miniature Accelerometer) were slightly better than a low-passed voice (at 200 Hz) in terms of number of periods detected by SEARP. Overall statistical results of f_0 distribution, however, did not differ significantly between the two methods. Severe low-pass or contact microphone voice data, however, are obviously not appropriate for pause-time analysis.

For any computer method to find daily and practical applications by clinicians, ease of operation is of the utmost importance. Thus, extensive on-line, machine-user interaction should be avoided. In addition, the analysis results should be available to the clinician either immediately or with minimal time lag and should be easy to interpret. From these considerations, program SEARP appears to have a potential for clinical applications. Once speech signals are digitized, many time-domain descriptions of speech are automatically produced without any user intervention. Effort to implement this analysis system in a clinical environment has been recently initiated at our laboratory.

SUMMARY

In summary, this chapter reviewed some approaches to early detection of laryngeal pathologies through acoustic analysis and discussed computer-assisted aerodynamic and acoustic analysis of alaryngeal speech conducted by this author. Because primary focus of the discussion was computer applications for alaryngeal speech analysis, specific mathematical techniques of general speech analysis and interactive systems for other disorder areas

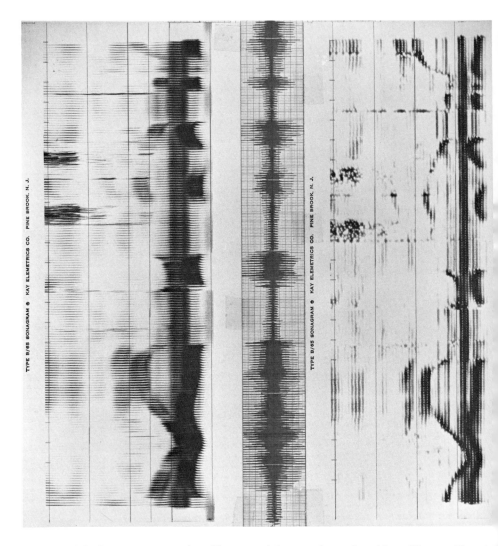

Figure 2-5. Spectrograms and oscillogram of the speech produced by a Western Electric artificial larynx.

were not discussed (Nickerson, Kalikow, and Stevens 1976; Levitt 1972; Boothroyd et al. 1975). Likewise, no mention was made of some special purpose hardware for f_0 analysis (such as Visi-Pitch® by Kay) intensity and pause analyzers, nor on the Sondhi

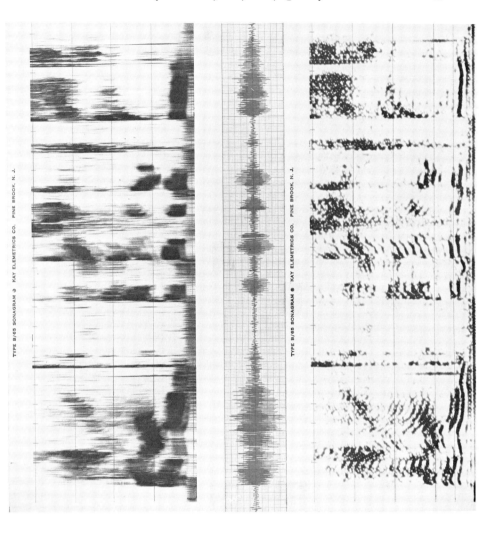

Figure 2-6. Spectrograms and oscillogram of a voice sample from the parabuccal speech.

Reflectionless Tube approach of sound-source analysis. Clearly, feasibility of both computer methods and analog methods should be rigorously explored in order to enhance diagnostic, rehabilitative, and evaluative procedures for laryngectomized individuals.

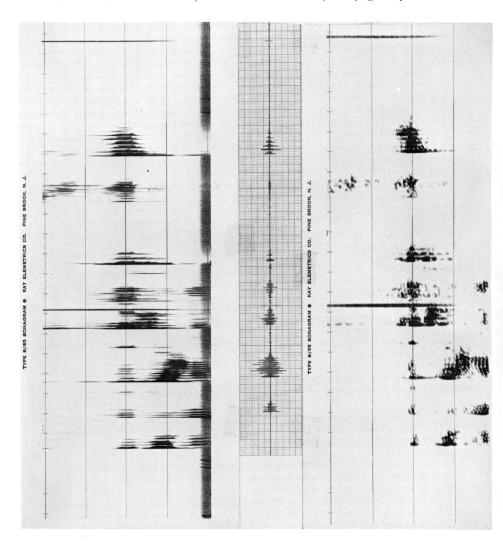

Figure 2-7. Spectrograms and oscillogram of a voice sample from the glossopharyngeal speech.

REFERENCES

Atal, B.S., and Hanauer, S.L.: Speech analysis and synthesis by linear prediction of the speech wave. *J Acoust Soc Am, 50*:637-655, 1971.

Atal, B.S., and Schroeder, M.R.: Predictive coding of speech signals. In Kohasi (Ed.): *Reports of the 6th International Congress on Acoustics*, 1968.

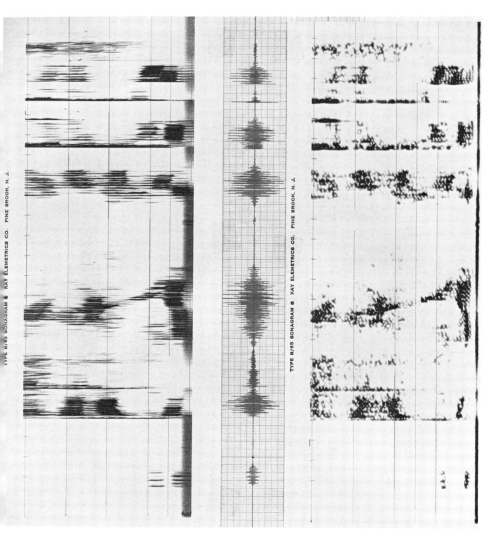

Figure 2-8. Spectrograms and oscillogram of a voice sample from the esophageal speech.

Beckett, R.L.: Pitch perturbation as a function of subjective vocal constriction. *Fonia Phoniatr, 21*:416-425, 1969.

Boothroyd, A., Archambault, P., Adams, R.E., and Storm, R.D.: Use of a computer-based system of speech analysis and display in a remedial speech program for deaf children. *Volta Review, 77*:178-193, 1975.

Bowler, N.W. A fundamental frequency analysis of harsh vocal quality. *Speech Monographs, 31*:128-134, 1964.

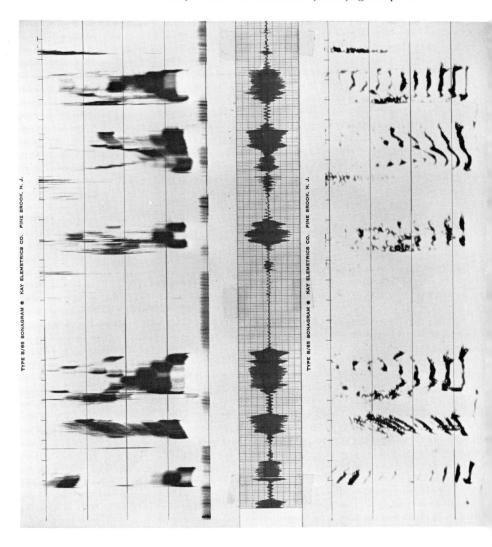

Figure 2-9. Spectrograms and oscillogram of a voice sample from the parabuccal speech

Cooke, P.A., and Horii, Y. *Respirometric Relationships Between Normal and Whispered Productions at Various Levels of Vocal Effort.* A paper presented at the 1975 Annual Meeting of the American Speech and Hearing Association, Washington, D.C., 1975.

Crystal, T.H., Montgomery, W.W., Jackson, C.L., and Johnson, N. *Methodology and Results on Laryngeal Disorder Detection through Speech Analysis.*

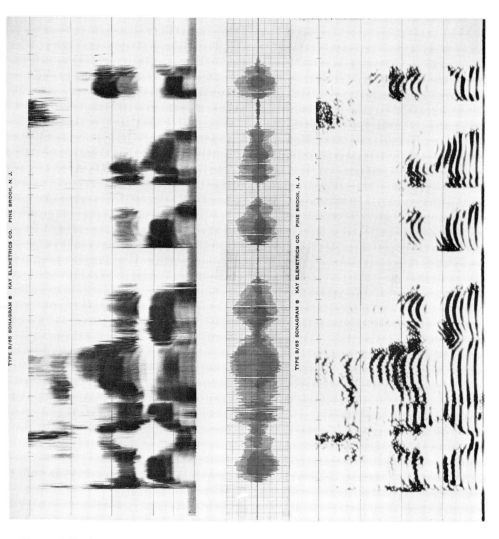

Figure 2-10. Spectrograms and oscillogram of a voice sample from the larynxophone artificial larynx speech.

Final Report, Contract PH-86-68-192 dated June 5, 1970. Signatron, Inc., Lexington, Massachusetts.

Davis, S.B.: Computer evaluation of laryngeal pathology based on inverse filtering of speech. *SCRL Monograph,* No. 13, 1976.

Deal, R.E., and Emanuel, F.W.: Some waveform and spectral features of vowel roughness. *J Speech Hear Res, 21*:250-264, 1978.

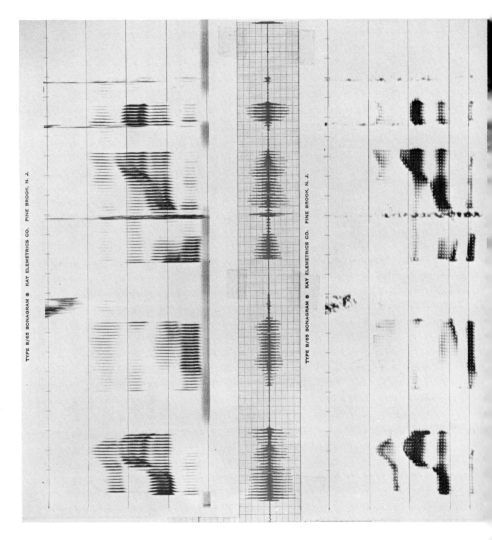

Figure 2-11. Spectrograms and oscillogram of a voice sample from the Pipa di Tichioi artificial larynx speech.

Denes, P.B.: On-line computers for speech research. *IEEE Trans Audio, 18*(4): 418-425, 1970.

Emanuel, F.W., Lively, M.A., and McCoy, J.F. Spectral noise levels and roughness ratings for vowels produced by males and females. *Folia Phoniatr., 25*: 110-120, 1973.

Gold, B.: Computer program for pitch extraction. *J Acoust Soc Am, 34*:916-921, 1962.

Hecker, M., and Kreul, E.J.: Descriptions of the speech of patients with cancer of the vocal folds. Part I: Measures of fundamental frequency. *J Acoust Soc Am, 49*:1275-1282, 1971.

Henke, W.L.: Speech and audio computer-aided examination and analysis facility. *Quart Prog Rep Lab Electron*, MIT, *95*:69-73, 1969.

Hiki, S., Imaizumi, S., Hirano, M., Matsushita, H., and Kakita, Y.: Acoustical analysis for voice disorders. *Conference Record, 1976 IEEE International Conference on Acoustics, Speech and Signal Processing.* Rome, New York: Canterbury Press, 1976.

Hollien, H., Michel, J., and Doherty, E.T.: A method for analyzing vocal jitter in sustained phonation. *J Phonetics, 1*:85-91, 1973.

Horii, Y.: Some statistical characteristics of voice fundamental frequency during oral reading. *J Speech Hear Res, 18*:192-201, 1975.

_____:Fundamental frequency perturbation observed in sustained phonation. *J Speech Hear Res, 22*:5-19, 1979.

_____: Vocal shimmer in sustained phonation. *J Speech Hear Res, 23*:202-209, 1980.

Horii, Y., and Cooke, P.A.: Some airflow, volume, and duration characteristics of oral reading. *J Speech Hear Res, 21*:470-481, 1978.

Horii, Y., and Hughes, G.W.: Speech analysis by computer. *Proceedings of the National Electronics Conference, 27*:74-79, 1972.

Isshiki, N.: Regulatory mechanism of voice intensity variation. *J Speech Hear Res, 7*:17-29, 1964.

Isshiki, N., Yanagihara, N., and Morimoto, M. Approach to objective diagnosis of hoarseness. *Folia Phoniatr, 18*:393-400, 1966.

Itakura, F., and Saito, S. Analysis synthesis telephony based upon the maximum likelihood method. *Conference Reports, 6th International Congress on Acoustics*, Kohasi (Ed.), Tokyo, 1968.

Iwata, S., and Von Leden, H.: Voice prints in laryngeal disease. Chicago: *Arch Otolaryngol, 91*(4), 346-351, 1970.

Jacob, L.: "A Normative Study of Laryngeal Jitter." Unpublished Master's Thesis, University of Kansas, 1968.

Kitajima, K.: An analysis of pitch perturbation in normal and pathologic voices. *Practica Otol, 66*:1195-1213, 1973.

Kitajima, K., and Gould, W.J.: Vocal shimmer in sustained phonation of normal and pathologic voice. *Ann Otol Rhinol Laryngol, 85*:377-381, 1976.

Koike, Y.: Vowel amplitude modulations in patients with laryngeal diseases. *J Acoust Soc Am, 45*:839-844, 1969.

_____: Application of some acoustic measures for the evaluation of laryngeal dysfunction. *Studia Phonologica, 7*:17-23, 1973.

Koike, Y., and Markel, J.D.: Application of inverse filtering for detecting laryngeal pathology. *Ann Otol Rhinol Laryngol, 84*:117-124, 1975.

Levitt, H.: Acoustic analysis of deaf speech using digital processing techniques. *IEEE Trans Audio Electro-Acoustics, AU-20*:35-41, 1972.

Lieberman, P.: Perturbations in vocal pitch. *J Acoust Soc Am, 33*:597-602, 1961.

_____:Some acoustic measures of the fundamental periodicity of normal and pathologic larynges. *J Acoust Soc Am, 35*:344-353, 1963.

Lieberman, P., and Michaels, S.B.: Some aspects of fundamental frequency and envelope amplitude as related to the emotional content of speech. *J Acoust Soc Am, 34*:922-927, 1962.

Makhoul, J.I., and Wolf, J.J.: Linear prediction and the spectral analysis of speech. *BBN Report 2304.* Cambridge, Massachusetts, Bolt, Beranek and Newman, Inc., 1972.

Markel, J.D., and Gray, A.H., Jr.: On autocorrelation equations as applied to speech analysis. *IEEE Trans Audio and Electroacoustics, AV-20:*69-79, 1973.

Mermelstein, P.: Computer-generated spectrogram displays for on-line speech research. *IEEE Trans Audio Electroacoustics, AV-19*(1):44-47, 1971.

Moore, P., and Von Leden, H.: Dynamic variations of the vibratory pattern in the normal larynx. *Folia Phoniatr, 10:*205-238, 1958.

Moore, P.G., and Thompson, C.: Comments on physiology of hoarseness. *Arch Otolaryngol, 81:*97-102, 1965.

Mysak, E.D.: Pitch and duration characteristics of older males. *J Speech Hear Res, 2:*46-54, 1959.

Nickerson, R.S., Kalikow, D.N., and Stevens, K.N. Computer-aided speech training for the deaf. *J Speech Hear Dis, 41:*120-132, 1976.

Noll, M.A.: Short-time spectrum and "cepstrum" techniques for vocal-pitch detection. *J Acoust Soc Am*, 36:296-302, 1964.

Oppenheim, A.V.: Speech spectrograms using the Fast Fourier Transform. *IEEE Spectrum, 7*(8):57-62, 1970.

Ramig, L., Ringel, R.L, and Horii, Y.: The voice characteristics of physically fit and unfit adult males, in press.

Schafer, R.W., and Rabiner, L.R.: System for automatic formant analysis of voiced speech. *J Acoust Soc Am, 47*:634-648, 1970.

Scripture, E.W.: *Researches in experimental phonetics: The study of speech curves.* Washington, D.C.: Carnegie Institute, 1906.

Shipp, T., and McGlone, R.L. Laryngeal dynamics associated with voice frequency change. *J Speech Hear Res, 14:*761-768, 1971.

Simon, C.: The variability of consecutive wave lengths in vocal and instrumental sounds. *Psychological Monographs, 36:*41-83, 1927.

Smith, B.E.: "Vocal Roughness and Jitter Characteristics of Selected Esophageal Vowels." Unpublished M.S. thesis, Purdue University, August, 1976.

Smith, W.R., and Lieberman, P.: Computer diagnosis of laryngeal lesion. *Comput Biomed Res 2*:291-303, 1969.

Snidecor, J.C., and Isshiki, N.: Air volume and airflow relationships of six male esophageal speakers. *J Speech Hear Dis, 30:*206-216, 1965.

Sorenson, D.N., and Horii, Y. The voice characteristics of smokers and non-smokers, in press.

Stevens, K.N., Kalikow, D.N., and Willemain, T.R. A miniature accelerometer for detecting glottal waveforms and nasalization. *J Speech Hear Res, 18*: 594-599, 1975.

Von Leden, H., and Koike, Y.: Detection of laryngeal disease by computer technique. *Arch Otolaryngol, 91*:3-10, 1970.

Von Leden, H., Moore, P., and Timake, R.: Laryngeal vibrations: Measurements of the glottal wave. Part III. The pathologic larynx. *AMA Arch Otolaryngol, 71*:16-35, 44, 1960.

Wakita, H.: Estimation of the vocal-tract shape by optimal inverse filtering and acoustic/articulatory conversion methods. *SCRL Monograph*, No. 9, 1972.

Weinberg, B., Dexter, R., and Horii, Y. Selected speech and fundamental frequency characteristics of patients with acromegaly. *J Speech Hear Dis, 40*: 253-259, 1975.

Weinberg, B., Shedd, D.P., and Horii, Y. Reed-fistula speech following pharyngolaryngectomy. *J Speech Hear Disord, 43*:401-413, 1978.

Wilcox, K.A., and Horii, Y.: Age and changes in vocal jitter. *J Gerontol, 35*:194-198, 1980.

Yanagihara, N.: Hoarseness: Investigation of the physiological mechanisms. *Ann Otol Rhinol Laryngol, 76*:472-488, 1967a.

————: Significance of harmonic changes and noise components in hoarseness. *J Speech Hear Res., 10*:531-541, 1967b.

Zemlin, W.R.: "A Comparison of the Periodic Function of Vocal Fold Vibration in a Multiple Sclerosis and a Normal Population." Unpublished Ph.D. thesis, University of Minnesota, 1962.

Zlatin-Laufer, M., and Horii, Y.: Fundamental frequency characteristics of infant non-distress vocalization during the first twenty-four weeks. *J Child Lang, 4*:171-184, 1977.

Chapter 3

ACOUSTIC CHARACTERISTICS OF EXCITATION SIGNAL FOR ALARYNGEAL SPEECH

SATOSHI IMAIZUMI, YASUO KOIKE AND TOSHIO MONJU

ABSTRACT

A comparative study of some acoustic characteristics of four kinds of alaryngeal speech and normal speech was carried out by using a computer analysis system and a sound spectrograph.

From the voice of a superior esophageal speaker, a regular periodical excitation signal comparable to the glottal volume velocity waveform for normal speaker's voice was extracted. It was observed that this signal contains a considerable amount of perturbation both in the fundamental frequency and in the amplitude, but not necessarily a large amount of noise components. Three distinctive accentuation types of Japanese two-mora words could be produced by this speaker.

The excitation signal extracted from the voice of a nonsuperior esophageal speaker was found to contain a large amount of noise components. The accentuation types spoken by this speaker could not be discriminated.

The perturbation in the fundamental frequency of the voice of a speaker using an electroartificial larynx was so small that the speech sounded very monotonous. It was difficult to discriminate each type of accentuation and to discriminate unvoiced sounds from voiced sounds produced by this speaker.

The excitation signal for a speaker using a Tokyo artificial larynx mostly resembled that of the normal speaker. The accentuation types could be pronounced correctly. However, it was difficult for this speaker to pronounce the unvoiced sounds clearly.

78

INTRODUCTION

THE ELECTROACOUSTIC INVESTIGATIONS of laryngectomee speech have widely been carried out with respect
to voice quality, supra-segmental features, and segmental features
by many researchers. It has been shown that the voice quality of
esophageal speech is characterized by very low fundamental
frequency, highly restricted variable range of the fundamental
frequency, monotonous sound, and a large amount of fluctuation
in the fundamental frequency etc. (Bennett and Weinberg 1973;
Filter and Hyman 1975; Curry 1977; Smith et al. 1978). The voice
quality of some kinds of artificial larynges has been shown to be
characterized by a very slow speaking rate, mechanical and
monotonous sound, and very low fundamental frequency (Bennett
and Weinberg 1973).

As for the supra-segmental features, it was indicated that some
Japanese esophageal speakers could pronounce Japanese two-
syllable word accentuation types correctly (Koike, Iwai, and
Morimoto 1975). Furthermore, it was shown that the voice onset
time and vowel duration of esophageal speech were different
from those of normal speech (Christensen and Weinberg 1976;
Christensen, Weinberg, and Alfonso 1978) and the intelligibility
score was very low—about 36 percent for esophageal speech
(Nichols 1976a, 1976b, 1977).

Some results of these investigations should be evaluated more
quantitatively, in order to elucidate the limitation of laryngectomee speech. The electroacoustic correlations, which generate
the characteristic sound of laryngectomee speech, can be measured
quantitatively with our computer evaluation system (Imaizumi
et al. 1980). The acoustic characteristics of excitation signal
for alaryngeal speech such as the amount of perturbation in the
fundamental frequency and in the amplitude, the amount of
noise components, and some fine features of glottal volume
velocity waveform are discussed quantitatively in this chapter.
The effects of these characteristics of some supra-segmental and
segmental features are also discussed.

EXPERIMENTAL PROCEDURE

Four kinds of laryngectomee speech were used as typical examples; that is, speech sounds uttered by a superior esophageal speaker (age 52, male), a nonsuperior esophageal speaker (age 61, male), a speaker (age 78, male) using an artificial electrolarynx (Aurex Neovox®), and one more speaker (age 69, male) using a Tokyo artificial larynx (Tapia-type 1 made by M. Okumura). A normal speech (age 30, male) was also employed for control.

Each speaker spoke five Japanese vowels and one kind of test sentence. These speech signals were recorded on a high-fidelity tape recorder (Teac A-4300). The vowel /ɛ/ signals were analyzed by the computer evaluation system mentioned above. The test sentences were analyzed with a sound spectrograph (Rion SG-07).

Figure 3-1 shows the block diagram of the computer evaluation system, which is composed of two parts. One is based on an autocorrelation analysis method with a long-time window (Davis 1976), and the other on a covariance method with a short-time window (Wong 1979). These are the methods used in linear prediction of speech (Markel and Gray 1976).

The gross characteristics of voices, such as the amount of perturbation in the fundamental frequency and in the amplitude, or the amount of noise components, can be extracted with the former. With the latter, some fine characteristics such as the irregularity in the glottal volume velocity waveform can be computed.

CHARACTERISTICS OF THE RESIDUE SIGNAL

Figure 3-2 shows the speech waveform and the residue wave-

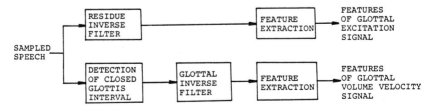

Figure 3-1. Computer system for the evaluation of laryngeal function.

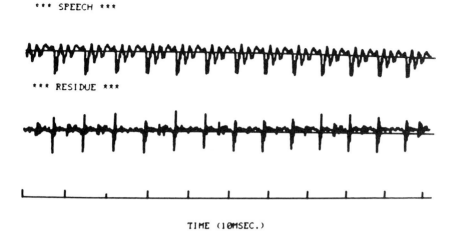

••• SPEECH •••

••• RESIDUE •••

TIME (10MSEC.)

Figure 3-2. Speech waveform and residue waveform of normal speech.

form extracted by the autocorrelation analysis from vowel /ε/ uttered by the normal speaker. It is observed that the residue signal is pulse-like in nature, and it indicates the pitch periods and the amplitude of the vocal-folds vibration. In this figure it is shown that there is a small amount of perturbation, both in the fundamental frequency and in the amplitude, and also a small amount of noise component in the normal voice.

These characteristics can be evaluated quantitatively by such parameters as Pitch Perturbation Quotient (PPQ), Amplitude Perturbation Quotient (APQ), and Coefficient of Excess (EX), which are extracted by the computer evaluation system. PPQ and APQ indicate the magnitude of perturbation in the fundamental frequency and in the amplitude of voice, respectively. These parameters were determined after Koike (1969, 1973). EX indicates the smallness of noise components defined after Davis (1976).

For the normal voice shown in Figure 3-2, PPQ was 0.003, APQ was 0.127, and EX was 18.61, respectively.

Figure 3-3 shows the speech waveform and residue waveform for the superior esophageal speech. The amount of perturbation in the fundamental frequency (PPQ = 0.127) and in the amplitude (APQ = 0.706) were very large; however, the amount of noise components were not so large (EX = 11.49). It was ascertained

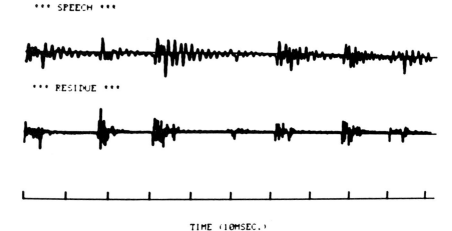

Figure 3-3. Speech waveform and residue waveform of superior esophageal speech.

based on synthetic speech (Imaizumi and Hiki 1978) that these large amounts of perturbation, both in the fundamental frequency and in the amplitude, made the voice hoarse. It can be seen that the fundamental frequency is very low, about 78 Hz (*see* Fig. 3-3).

Figure 3-4 illustrates the speech waveform and residue waveform for the nonsuperior esophageal speech. The epoch and amplitude of pulses corresponding to the vibration of the vocal folds cannot be observed, obviously. There is a large amount of perturbation both in the fundamental frequency (PPQ = 0.101) and in the amplitude (APQ = 0.281) and, importantly, a large amount of noise component is observed (EX = 5.99). It is believed that the large amount of noise component gives the speech a "breathy" sound. The main difference in the residue signal between the superior and the nonsuperior esophageal speech was the amount of noise components. This difference might originate from the difference of vibration mode of the pseudoglottis.

In Figure 3-5, the speech waveform and the residue waveform for the speech uttered, using the artificial electrolarynx, is shown. The linear-prediction analysis model does not fit this speech strictly, because the sound is radiated not only from the mouth but also directly from the vibrator. And the way of excitation of the vocal tract is very different from that in the normal speaker, since the excitation signal is transmitted to the vocal tract through the skin. This problem might be very complicated. However, in Figure 3-5 it can be seen from the speech waveform

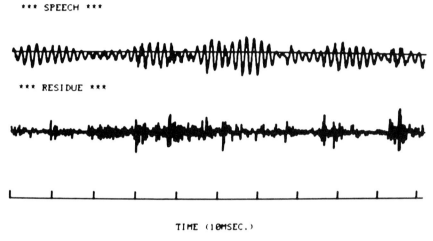

Figure 3-4. Speech waveform and residue waveform of nonsuperior esophageal speech.

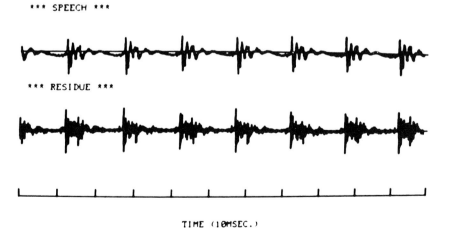

Figure 3-5. Speech waveform and residue waveform of artificial electrolarynx speech.

that the amount of perturbation in the fundamental frequency is very small (PPQ was 0.001 in trial calculation); also the noise component is very small (EX = 11.99). It was ascertained based on synthetic speech that these characteristics make the speech mechanical.

The speech waveform and residue waveform for the speech uttered using a Tokyo artificial larynx may be seen in Figure 3-6. Strictly speaking, this kind of speech is not fitted to the linear-prediction analysis model, because of the tube inserted into the mouth to produce the excitation signal. However, the approximation error for this kind of speech might not be so large as the one for the speech using an artificial electrolarynx.

The amount of perturbation in the fundamental frequency (PPQ = 0.039), in the amplitude (APQ = 0.164), and in the amount of noise components (EX = 12.00) were somewhat larger than those of the normal speech, but smaller than those of the two kinds of esophageal speech. Among these four kinds of laryngectomee speech, the voice quality of the speech uttered, using the Tokyo artificial larynx, most closely resembled the normal one.

CHARACTERISTICS OF GLOTTAL VOLUME VELOCITY WAVEFORM

The residue signal should be considered as an excitation signal of a linear model simulating the speech-production system, including all the characteristics of the vocal cords vibration, the vocal-tract transmission, and the lip radiation. In contrast, the waveform, extracted from the speech waveform by subtracting only the characteristics of the vocal-tract transmission and the lip radiation, should be considered as a waveform corresponding to the glottal volume velocity waveform. Such a signal could be extracted by using glottal inverse filtering (Hiki et al. 1976; Wong, Markel, and Gray 1979). This signal contains some fine characteristics of the glottal volume velocity waveform.

Figure 3-7 shows the speech waveform and the extracted glottal volume velocity waveform of the normal speech. In this figure, a periodical triangular waveform corresponding to the vibration of the vocal cords can be observed; a regular and repetitive closed phase is clearly observed.

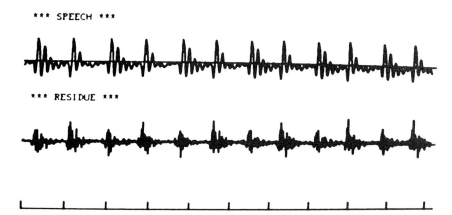

*** SPEECH ***

*** RESIDUE ***

TIME (10MSEC.)

Figure 3-6. Speech waveform and residue waveform of speech with a Tokyo artificial larynx.

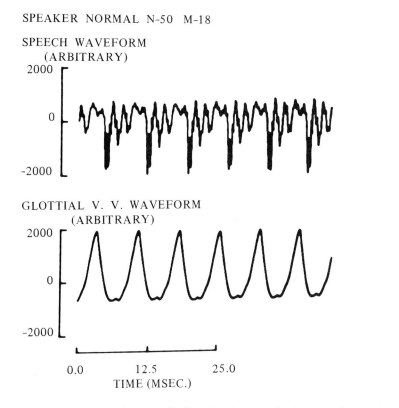

SPEAKER NORMAL N-50 M-18

SPEECH WAVEFORM
(ARBITRARY)

GLOTTIAL V. V. WAVEFORM
(ARBITRARY)

TIME (MSEC.)

Figure 3-7. Speech waveform and glottal volume velocity waveform of normal speech.

In the next illustration the speech waveform and the waveform corresponding to the glottal volume velocity waveform of the superior esophageal speech can be seen. Also, this signal is very different from that of the normal speech (*see* Figure 3-8).

The excitation signal extracted from the nonsuperior esophageal speech was very noisy, and no periodical pulse-like triangular waveform could be observed.

Figure 3-9 illustrates the speech waveform and the waveform corresponding to the glottal volume velocity waveform extracted from the speech uttered using the Tokyo artificial larynx. It is clearly evident that this signal has a regularly periodic series of pulse-like triangular waveform and very much resembles that of normal speech.

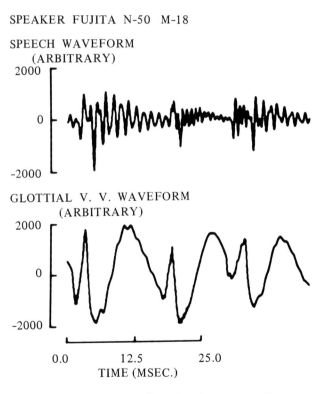

Figure 3-8. Speech waveform and a signal corresponding to the glottal volume velocity waveform of a superior esophageal speech.

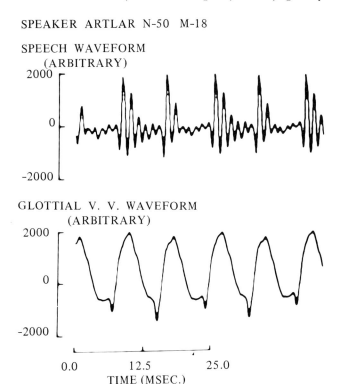

SPEAKER ARTLAR N-50 M-18

Figure 3-9. Speech waveform and a signal corresponding to the glottal volume velocity waveform of a speech using a Tokyo artificial larynx.

THE EFFECTS OF ACOUSTIC CHARACTERISTICS ON THE SUPRA-SEGMENTAL FEATURES

The acoustic characteristics of the excitation signal may have some effects on the supra-segmental and segmental features. In order to clarify these effects, we used here a sentence "Korewa (something) desu," which means that "this is a (something)," after Koike, Iwai, and Morimoto (1975). Three two-mora nouns, as shown in Table 3-I, and some other words for control were inserted in lieu of "something." In other words, the subjects spoke like "Korewa hashi desu," etc., in a random order in Kansai dialect of Japanese. These speech signals were recorded on the high-fidelity tape recorder and analyzed with the sound spectro-

Table 3-I. Three Accentuation Types of Japanese Two-Mora Words

Type	Word	Pitch Pattern	Meaning
A	/ha ʃ i/		an edge
B	/ha ʃ i/		a bridge
C	/ha ʃ i/		chopsticks

graph. The test words, which were inserted into the test sentence, had some particular characteristics. The words A, B, and C in Table 3-I have the same phonemic structure and are discriminated from each other only by their supra-segmental features or prosodic patterns. Table 3-I also illustrates the prosodic patterns of Japanese two-mora nouns. The test word B in Table 3-I (which means a bridge) has a falling intonation. The words A and C have a rising tone and are distinguished from each other by another clue. The differences of the prosodic patterns between the words A and B are very clear, so only the contrasts between A and B will be discussed hereafter.

In Figure 3-10, two kinds of sound spectrograms of the normal speech are shown. The upper ones are the patterns produced with a narrow-band filter, and the others are the amplitude displays. From both kinds of the sound spectrograms, the difference between two kinds of the prosodic patterns can be clearly distinguished. One pattern has a rising tone and the other, a falling one. And, furthermore, some characteristic noise components corresponding to the consonants /h/ and / ʃ / of /haʃ i/ are clearly observed.

The patterns and the amplitude displays for the superior esophageal speech are seen in Figure 3-11. These patterns were produced with a wide-band filter. The pitch information could not be observed with the narrow-band filter, since the fundamental frequency was too low. The fundamental periods can be observed at some durations corresponding to the vowels /ɑ/ or /i/. However, this speech seems noisy due to the large amount of

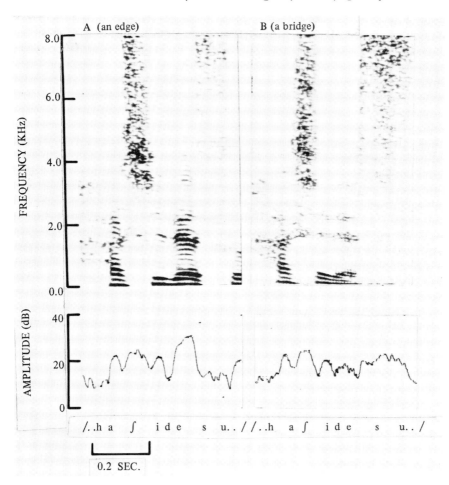

Figure 3-10. Sound spectrograms of normal speech.

perturbation both in the fundamental frequency and in the amplitude. The difference of each prosodic pattern cannot be observed from the spectrum, but it can be observed from the amplitude displays. This speaker could pronounce each prosodic pattern distinguishably. Some characteristic noise components cannot be observed at the duration corresponding to the consonant /h/, but it can be observed at the duration corresponding to the consonant / ʃ /.

For the nonsuperior esophageal speech, neither the difference

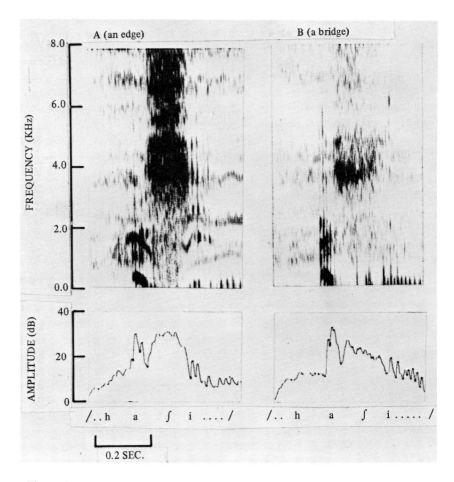

Figure 3-11. Sound spectrograms of a superior esophageal speech.

of each prosodic pattern, nor the characteristic harmonic components corresponding to the vowels /ɑ/ or /i/ could be observed. It was difficult to distinguish between the voiced and unvoiced duration of /hɑ ʃ i/ based on any sound spectrograms of this speech, because of the great amount of noise components. For the speech uttered using the artificial electrolarynx, unvoiced duration, which should appear in normal pronounciation of /ha ʃ i/, could not be observed, and the fundamental frequency was strictly constant. The amplitude was changed according to the opening area of the lips, and therefore, it was difficult for this speaker to pronounce the prosodic patterns distinguishably. Also it was difficult to discriminate the unvoiced sounds from the voiced sounds pronounced by this speaker.

Figure 3-12 shows the patterns and the amplitude displays of the speech uttered using the Tokyo artificial larynx. The difference of each prosodic pattern could be distinguished clearly from both of them; however, no unvoiced duration could be observed. The consonant /h/ could not be pronounced clearly. Some characteristic noise components at a higher-frequency range appeared at the segment corresponding to the consonant / ʃ /. Therefore, this speaker pronounced something like /ɑzi/, instead

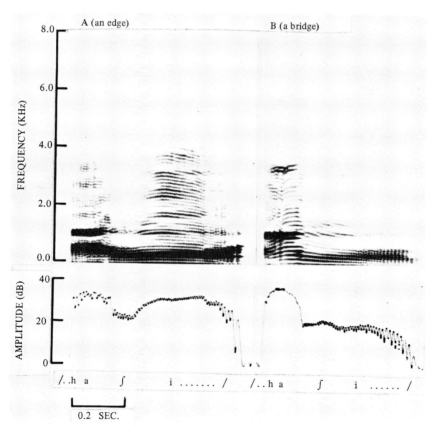

Figure 3-12. Sound spectrograms of speech with a Tokyo artificial larynx.

of /hɯ ʃ i/, actually. It can be seen from Figure 3-12 that the
speaking rate of this speaker was very slow.

DISCUSSION

Some acoustic characteristics of four kinds of laryngectomee
speech and a normal speech for control were compared quantitatively.

In the normal speech, it was shown that the amount of
perturbation both in the fundamental frequency and in the
amplitude were not so large, and the amount of noise components
was small. The glottal volume velocity waveform was a regular
and periodic series of pulse-like triangular waveforms; the
closed phase was clearly observed. Three accentuation types of
Japanese two-mora words were pronounced correctly.

In the superior esophageal speech, a regular and periodic
excitation signal comparable to the glottal volume velocity
waveform for the normal speaker's voice could be observed.
However, this signal was seen to contain a considerable amount
of perturbation both in the fundamental frequency and in the
amplitude. It is thought that these characteristics make the
speech hoarse. The amount of noise components was not large.
Three accentuation types of Japanese two-mora words could be
pronounced discriminatively by this speaker; however, this
speaker could not distinguish these accentuation types as clearly
as the normal speaker, because of the great amount of perturbation both in the fundamental frequency and in the amplitude.
The glottal consonant /h/ could not be uttered clearly, and the
fundamental frequency was very low.

In the nonsuperior esophageal speech, the extracted excitation
signal contained a large amount of noise components; no
periodic series of a pulse-like triangular waveform could be
extracted. This speaker could not produce the voiced sounds
clearly, but he could pronounce the accentuation types distinguishably.

For the speech uttered using the artificial electrolarynx, the
fundamental frequency was so strictly constant that the speech
sounded very monotonous and mechanical. The noise components were not so large, and it was difficult for this speaker to

produce the unvoiced sounds clearly and to pronounce the accentuation types correctly.

For the speech using the Tokyo artificial larynx, the excitation signal mostly resembled that of normal speech. The amount of perturbation both in the fundamental frequency and in the amplitude were larger than those of the speech uttered using the artificial electrolarynx, but smaller than those of the two kinds of esophageal speech; therefore, the voice quality was very natural. The accentuation types were pronounced discriminatively; however, it was difficult for this speaker to pronounce the unvoiced sounds clearly.

This investigation was limited to some typical examples, and these results should be generalized by investigating more examples. We are making plans to investigate the mechanism of voice production, or vibration mechanism of pseudoglottis for laryngectomee speakers, by means of physiological observation. Also, we are going to carry out some more comparative studies between physiological and electroacoustical characteristics to elucidate the limitation of laryngectomee speech in order to advance rehabilitation for the handicapped.

REFERENCES

Bennett, S., and Weinberg, B.: Acceptability ratings of normal, esophageal, and artificial laryngeal speech. *J Speech Hear Res*, 16:605, 1973.

Christensen, J.M., and Weinberg, B.: Vowel duration characteristics of esophageal speech. *J Speech Hear Res*, 19:678, 1976.

Christensen, J.M., Weinberg, B., and Alfonso, P.J.: Productive voice onset time characteristics of esophageal speech. *J Speech Hear Res*, 21:56, 1978.

Curry, E.T.: Some acoustical aspects of alaryngeal speech. *Ear Nose Throat J*, 56:26, 1977.

Davis, S.B.: *Computer evaluation of laryngeal pathology based on inverse filtering of speech (SCRL MONOGRAPH No. 13)*. Santa Barbara, Speech Communication Research Laboratory, 1976.

Filter, M.D., and Hyman, M.: Relationship of acoustic parameters and perceptual ratings of esophageal speech. *Percept Mot Skills*, 40:63, 1975.

Hiki, S., Imaizumi, S., Hirano, M., Matsushita, M., and Kakita, Y.: Acoustical analysis of voice disorders. *Conference Record, 1976 IEEE Int. Conf. Acoust. Speech Sig. Proc.*, 613, 1976.

Imaizumi, S., and Hiki, S.: Scaling the perceptual quality of pathological voice by the use of synthetic speech. *J Acoust Soc Am, 64, Suppl. 1*:52, 1978.

Imaizumi, S., Ohta, F., Koike, Y., Moniu, T., Yonekawa, H., and Abe, H.: Evaluation of laryngeal function by acoustic analysis. *Jpn. Acoust. Soc., Conference Record on Speech S79-65 (1980-2):*497, 1980 (in Japanese).

Koike, Y.: Vowel amplitude modulations in patients with laryngeal diseases. *J Acoust Soc Am, 45:*839, 1969.

———: Application of some acoustic measures for the evaluation of laryngeal dysfunction. *Studia Phonologica, 7:*17, 1973.

Koike, Y., Iwai, H., and Morimoto, M.: Restoration of voice after laryngeal surgeries. *Laryngoscope, 85:*4, 1975.

Markel, J.D., and Gray, A.H. Jr.: *Linear Prediction of Speech.* Berlin: Springer-Verlag, 1976.

Nichols, A.C.: Confusions in recognizing phonemes spoken by esophageal speakers: I. Initial consonants and clusters. *J Commun Disord, 9:*27, 1976a.

———: Confusions in recognizing phonemes spoken by esophageal speakers: II. Vowels and diphthongs. *J Commun Disord, 9:*247, 1976b.

———: Confusions in recognizing phonemes spoken by esophageal speakers: III. Terminal consonants and clusters. *J Commun Disord, 10:*285, 1977.

Smith, B.E., Weinberg, B., Feth, L.L., and Horii, Y.: Vocal roughness and jitter characteristics of vowels produced by esophageal speakers. *J Speech Hear Res, 21:*240, 1978.

Wong, D.Y., Markel, J.D., and Gray, A.H. Jr.: Least squares glottal inverse filtering from the acoustic speech waveform. *IEEE Trans. ASSP, ASSP-27, 4:* 350, 1979.

Chapter 4

ACOUSTIC ANALYSIS OF ARTIFICIAL ELECTRONIC LARYNX SPEECH

Howard B. Rothman

ABSTRACT

The research literature concerning neck-type artificial larynges is relatively sparse and, until recent years, has been primarily concerned with comparing artificial larynx speech with esophageal and normal speech. Partial responsibility for this lack of information derives from the past negative attitudes concerning the use of electronic devices by speech pathologists, physicians, and the International Association of Laryngectomees. Fortunately, these attitudes are changing, and many individuals working with laryngectomees are encouraging the development of both esophageal and electronic larynx speech. This is true, especially since recent investigations have shown that the acquisition of one mode of speech production does not interfere with or preclude the acquisition of the other mode of production.

Many studies have compared good and poor esophageal speakers, and this information has been used to establish standardized criteria for esophageal speech. However, there is virtually no information that compares good to poor electronic larynx speakers. Thus, there are relatively few usable data with which to establish standards and criteria for the evaluation of artificial larynx speech and for determining when to terminate treatment for speech purposes. Therefore, it is essential to determine the degree of speech proficiency, categorizing good and poor electronic larynx speakers before a comparison of their respective speech productions can be attempted.

This chapter presents the results of research conducted at the University of Florida's Institute for Advanced Study of the Communication Processes and the Gainesville Veterans Administration Medical Center. These studies provide information necessary for determining speech communication proficiency and the grouping of electronic larynx users into good and poor categories. Further, data will be presented concerning measurements of those parameters that served to define speech communication proficiency. These include: frequency range, intensity range, rate of speaking, fricative production, stop/consonant closure durations, and intensity variations within stop closures. Finally, implications for utilizing laboratory-type measurements in a clinical setting will be discussed.

A REVIEW OF THE LITERATURE concerning the speech of the laryngectomized will reveal a surprising lack of useful information concerning neck-placed artificial electronic larynges. Much of the literature that is available is concerned with comparing artificial larynx speech to esophageal or normal speech or discusses the controversy regarding the use of esophageal as opposed to artificial larynx speech. The paucity of investigative information on the electronic larynx and on speech produced with such a device is, indeed, surprising, especially when one considers that they have been available for almost forty years and are the most widely used of the artificial larynges.

Lauder (1968), Carter (1976), Goldstein (1976, 1978), and Berry (1978) have provided a review of the reasons for and against the use of an artificial larynx. The reasons most often encountered against the use of an artificial larynx are that it (1) is an unnecessary crutch; (2) interferes with the development of esophageal speech; (3) results in unintelligible and/or noisy speech; (4) requires the use of a hand; (5) involves a bulky and awkward instrument; (6) calls attention to an infirmity; (7) requires expensive maintenance; and (8) causes a person to be speechless if a breakdown occurs. The contention that use of an artificial larynx interferes with the development of esophageal speech is not true. The assertion that its use results in unintelligible and/or noisy speech is a specious one. Some artificial larynges are noisier than others, and all of them, when used properly, will enable a talker to produce speech that is quite intelligible and even relatively free of extraneous noise.

Reasons *for* the use of an artificial larynx include: (1) it is a psychological and economic necessity for the newly laryngectomized; (2) esophageal speech cannot be developed immediately after recovery from surgical trauma; (3) it is often more intelligible than esophageal speech in a variety of communication situations; (4) it is easily understood over the phone; (5) it enables a user to communicate more effectively in situations involving emotional stress; (6) it provides greater volume; (7) it permits prompt and immediate speech; (8) it is easily learned; (9) it can be used by individuals of advanced age and/or by individuals in poor health; (10) it can be used by those incapable of learning esophageal speech; and (11) there is no difficulty in using both esophageal and electro-laryngeal speech alternately (Carter 1976).

Perhaps the most persuasive reason for making an effective artificial larynx available to all laryngectomized individuals including those proficient in esophageal speech has been provided by Lauder (1970), who is a laryngectomee and a member of the Board of Directors, International Association of Laryngectomees. In his report, Lauder (1970) described three events involving laryngectomized patients in acute situations that precluded the use of esophageal speech at a particular time. One person had an attack of pancreatitis and could not communicate with a physician by telephone; a second had a draining hypopharyngeal fistula that exuded copious secretions at each attempt to inject air for esophageal speech; and the third had not developed esophageal speech and, therefore, could not communicate the fact that his wife was having a heart attack.

From the Lauder report, it is obvious that individuals who have acquired esophageal speech can experience difficulty in maintaining it under various conditions and situations, including psychological and physical stress and when they have colds and infections. Further, extensive surgery involving the esophagus, poor pharyngeal or esophageal stricture, extensive radiation, heart problems, hiatus hernia, emphysema, and other respiratory insufficiencies will curtail or preclude the use of esophageal speech communication.

As already stated, most of the research regarding laryngectomized speech has been concerned with comparisons between esophageal and artificial larynx speech intelligibility (Hyman 1955; Crouse 1962; McCroskey and Mulligan 1963; Shames, Font, and Matthews 1963; Bennett and Weinberg 1973; Goldstein 1974). With the exception of a few clinical reports and tests usually performed on a single speaker, there have been virtually no controlled investigations of artificial larynx speech. However,

Goldstein and Rothman (1976, 1978) have initiated a series of experiments that are designed to examine the acoustic character-istics of the various artificial larynges and the effects of their coupling to the tissues of the neck. The information that will ultimately derive from these investigations, coupled with data establishing standards for evaluating artificial larynx speech, will enable scientists and clinicians to develop criteria for comparing superior, good, and poor talkers and for determining when, and if, treatment should be terminated.

THE ARTIFICIAL ELECTRONIC LARYNX

Basically, there are two types of electrical artificial larynges: (1) the oral type that places the sound directly into the oral cavity through a tube; and (2) the throat type that is held against the neck and thereby transmits sound into the pharynx and mouth. This chapter will be concerned with the second type, i.e. the electronic, neck-placed artificial larynx.

The most widely used artificial larynges are, essentially, electromechanical vibrators, which excite the inner surface of the neck (or throat), thereby generating an acoustic signal through the opening of the oral cavity. The vibrational input is in the form of pulses where the pulse rate corresponds to the desired frequency characteristics of a male or female voice. Generally, the pulse width is on the order of a millisecond or less in order to produce vibratory acoustic responses in the kilohertz range. The Fourier series matching the pulse shape and width restricts the possible available frequency components. The acoustic output from the mouth is further determined by vocal-tract config-uration.

In order for these devices to be portable, they have a self-contained battery power supply. The power necessary to achieve pulse-peak vibration levels in order to overcome inefficiencies of the mechanical driver, as well as the mechanical loading of the skin tissue to which the driver is pressed, is high. However, for low pulse rates and small pulse widths, the power duty factor remains low enough to provide several hours of use with available batteries.

The devices now available (Lauder 1975; Lebrun 1973, and

Goode 1975) allow the patient to vary the location of application and to control the pressure at the driver face. The loading of the driver face is, in part, determined by the nature of the surrounding tissue. This configuration tends to generate significant amounts of airborne acoustic energy outside the neck as well as in the vocal cavity. Vibratory damping due to human tissue will reduce amplitudes away from the position of application. Nevertheless, some vibratory components will be transmitted throughout a portion of the cranial structure. This bone-conducted energy acts as a masking stimulus.

Attempts to improve the quality of the acoustic signal output of external prostheses are sometimes associated with a manually operated switch on the device that shifts the pulse rate. This switch evidently alters the central low-frequency components of the signal and, to a lesser extent, modifies the high-frequency response. Because of the frequency response of the ear of the patient or his listener, shifting to a higher pulse rate often is perceived as a slight increase in loudness of the voiced output. Although the intent of the pulse rate shift is to enable a speaker to approximate inflectional patterns, it is rarely used efficiently.

FACTORS AFFECTING SPEECH
COMMUNICATION PROFICIENCY

Any attempt at planning or initiating a treatment program involving the use of an artificial larynx or any attempt at determining speech communication proficiency with an artificial larynx should consider the following:

1. Most laryngectomees were normal speakers and would still be normal speakers for their age group, dialectal group, socioeconomic-educational status, and general health group if their larynges were not surgically removed.

2. Empirical observations have determined that a functional articulatory mechanism is often retained by laryngectomees after surgery. These observations, when restricted to users of electronic larynges, are supported by statements of Stetson (1937), Kallen (1934), and Morton (1973). Their conclusions are in agreement that problems affecting speech are related more to aerodynamics than to articulation.

Therefore, depending on the extent of surgery, differences in observed or measured speech communication proficiency may be related to conditions existing prior to the surgical removal of the larynx or to conditions not related to the laryngectomy.

Other factors that can affect speech communication proficiency are instructions for the introduction of acoustic and temporal distortions. For example, literature accompanying some of the available electronic larynges suggests that proper usage requires speaking slowly, elongating vowels and syllables, overemphasizing certain sounds, and using a staccato-like rhythm based on syllabic units. This approach can introduce amplitude and temporal distortions to the speech production process that, in turn, will tend to obscure or modify those parameters serving as perceptual cues for speech. This approach also is suggesting that an individual with a functional articulatory system and a long-term habituated speech pattern is being requested to change that pattern at a time when he is suffering emotional and physical trauma. Therefore, it appears that approaches to electronic larynx use tend to add artificial constraints to the speech signal over and above the artificiality inherent in the device itself.

If one accepts the contention that a functional articulatory system has been retained, the problem is that the source of voicing and airflow/pressure has been altered. Air no longer is directed from the lungs through the glottis and trachea into the oral cavity. Because of this, other means for increasing air pressure and airflow are necessary. The means utilized by most artificial larynx users is buccal air. Buccal air (i.e. air impounded within the oral cavity) can be effectively used for the production of stop, fricative, and affricate consonants.

DETERMINING SPEECH COMMUNICATION PROFICIENCY

In an effort to determine speech communication proficiency, Goldstein and Rothman (1976) recorded fifteen artificial larynx talkers who were reading eight C.I.D. Everyday Sentences. The recording process followed well-established procedures to insure that the recording itself would not become a variable affecting the data. Six experienced speech pathologists rated each talker's speech communication proficiency on a seven-point, equal-appearing interval scale, with one representing least proficient and seven representing most proficient. Ratings were based upon the speech pathologists' experience as to what constituted verbal communication proficiency. An inter-judge reliability of average ratings was 0.76, which indicated that they were using similar criteria in their judgments. The fifteen speakers were then grouped according to their averaged score into three equal groups. The group of the five highest-scoring talkers (with a mean proficiency rating of 6.33) and the group of the five lowest-scoring talkers (with a mean proficiency rating of 2.73) were then used for comparison. The difference between the two groups' mean proficiency ratings was significant at the 0.001 level.

All of the talkers used neck-placed, electronic artificial larynges. Seven used a Western Electric No. 5 device and three used an Aurex Neovox device. The average age of the poor talkers was five years greater than that of the good talkers. The poor talkers had, on the average, 1.6 less years of education. Average length of time from surgery was seven years. None of the talkers were involved with speech treatment at the time of their participation in this study. However, the poor talkers had an average of 1.2 more hours of speech treatment than did the good talkers.

The speech parameters of rate/duration, frequency range of the vibratory pulses produced by the electronic larynges, and intensity range were measured. Analysis of the data provided validation for the speech pathologists' grouping of the talkers. The data (as shown in Table 4-I) indicated the following:

1. RATE/DURATION

   Good talkers read a twelve-word sentence with a mean rate of 3.86 seconds (standard deviation of 0.36), as contrasted to the poor talkers' mean rate of 6.48 seconds (standard deviation of 2.23). The larger mean and standard deviation found for the poor talkers indicate an intra- and inter-group differential in the ability to coordinate electronic larynx activation/deactivation during the course of the sentence. Poor talkers tend to pause more often than good talkers. During the pause they also tend to deactivate (in effect, shut down) the device. These pauses would occur between phrase groups. Therefore, each phrase group within a long

Table 4-I. Mean and Standard Deviations for Speech Communication Proficiency Ratings for Two Groups of Electronic Larynx Talkers. Results of a Mann-Whitney U Test Indicate the Significance of the Differences Between the Two Groups.

	Proficiency Ratings*	Rate of Speaking†	Frequency Range‡
Poor Speakers			
Means	2.73	6.48	11.10
S.D.	0.87	2.23	3.42
Good Speakers			
Means	6.33	3.86	16.10
S.D.	0.28	0.36	2.48
Mann-Whitney U	0	1	3
P =	0.001	0.008	0.028

*On seven-point scale.
†Time to read 12 word sentence, in seconds.
‡In Hertz.

and a complex sentence would, in effect, be treated as a sentence initiation, and the long sentence becomes a series of short sentences.

2. FREQUENCY RANGE

Frequency range was obtained from a twelve-word sentence by using the paper readout of a Honeywell 1508A Visicorder®. The frequency ranges of the poor talkers varied from 6.61 to 15.32 Hz, with a mean range of 11.10 Hz and a standard deviation of 3.42. The good talkers varied frequency from 13.06 to 20.26, with a mean range of 16.10 Hz and a standard deviation of 2.48. Interestingly, the three talkers with the widest frequency range were using an Aurex Neovox, which does not have a pitch control. At a later date, frequency range measurements were obtained from a user of a Western Electric No. 5 (which has a variable pitch control) who was rated as a superior talker. This talker, using the Western Electric, typically varies pitch appropriately and in a manner similar to prelaryngectomee speech patterns by as much as 50 Hz within one sentence.

3. INTENSITY RANGE

Intensity ranges were obtained through a B & K Level

Recorder and the amplitude display of a Voice Identification Series 700 Spectrograph. Measurements from the B & K are in microvolts; in db from the spectrograph. This parameter was extremely difficult to measure and quantify from the data obtained from the group of poor talkers. Some of the poor talkers exhibited almost no change in intensity; others exhibited large and inappropriate fluctuations in intensity, while still others shut the device down during stop consonantal closures, voiceless fricatives, and pauses within a sentence or phrase group. In comparison, the good talkers maintained a more constant overall intensity level, with small, subtle changes used to indicate devoicing during stops, voiceless consonants, and pauses.

In any event, there are significant differences between the two groups that serve to categorize them as having either good or poor speech communication proficiency with an electronic larynx. Rate/duration and intensity were particularly significant in this regard. Many people focus on pitch as a significant parameter, though it is not. Even when available, most electronic larynx users do not use the variable pitch control, and it appears that listeners did not seem to rate it as a significant factor in determining proficiency.

How are pitch and intensity variations produced by the good users of the electronic larynx? The vibrating disc on the electronic larynges, which couples to the neck, is mechanically driven by a piston. Coupling pressure can be varied by increasing or decreasing the pressure of the device to the neck. Changes in pressure cause a change in the relationship between the disc and piston, which serves to increase or reduce the excursion of the piston. This, in turn, can affect frequency and intensity by (1) causing a differential loading effect on the electronics producing the pulse rate with which the piston is driven and thereby affecting frequency; and (2) causing piston movements to be damped or undamped, thereby reducing or increasing intensity.

One other variable served to distinguish the two groups; that variable was *extraneous noise*. Extraneous noise occurs when the electronic larynx is improperly coupled to the tissues of the neck. Good talkers will have no extraneous noises; poor talkers do.

ELECTRONIC LARYNX CHARACTERISTICS

The ideal electronic larynx should produce periodic energy at least throughout the speech range (i.e. up to approximately 4,000 Hz.) This frequency range would encompass spectral areas for vowel formants of men, women, and children. Further, the energy produced by the devices and transmitted through the tissues of the neck into the vocal tract should, then, be modulated by the vocal-tract resonances.

A spectral analysis was performed of the output of the Servox, Aurex Neovox, Western Electric No. 5, and Barts appliances under two conditions: coupled and uncoupled to neck tissue. Some exhibited energy distributed over a much wider range than others. For example, the Servox generated the smallest distribution of energy, and the Western Electric generated the widest distribution of energy. All of them showed spectral regions of energy concentration. The discussion below will focus on the maximized areas of energy. It should be noted that different models of each device will exhibit some variation in spectral output as well as in distribution of energy through the spectrum. Further, neck placement was not systematically controlled, since it is not controlled in circumstances of ordinary usage by a laryngectomee. Therefore, each device was coupled to the neck tissue on the basis of the talker determining that the device felt comfortable and produced good acoustic output.

When uncoupled from the tissue, the Servox (*see* Figure 4-1) generated strong energy between 100-300 Hz and 1000-4000 Hz. When coupled to tissue, (*see* Figure 4-2) the strongest energy was found between 770 and 1385 Hz. The Aurex Neovox, when uncoupled (*see* Figure 4-3) produced bands of maximized energy at 580-890 Hz, 1540-2310 Hz, 2460-2770 Hz, 3000-4460 Hz, and 4490-5845 Hz. When coupled (*see* Figure 4-4), the distribution changed to bands located between 500-1385 Hz, 2155-2615 Hz, and 3845-4230 Hz, with a weaker, contiguous band extending up to 4690 Hz. The Western Electric No. 5, when uncoupled (*see* Figure 4-5), produced the widest distribution of energy. These were located in bands between 70-385 Hz, 2000-2155 Hz, 3155-4000 Hz, 6000-6615 Hz, and 7000-7695 Hz. When coupled (*see* Figure 4-6), the energy bands were located between 615-1310 Hz,

1770-2615 Hz, 3385-3845 Hz, 4885-5460 Hz, and 5845-6310 Hz. The Barts vibrator's pulse output appears to be less damped than the others and, therefore, generates a less-discrete pulse and energy distribution. When uncoupled (*see* Figure 4-7), a strong band of energy was found between 810-1460 Hz. Contiguous with this band was an undifferentiated diffuse and less-intense band of energy up to 3230 Hz. When coupled to tissue (*see* Figure 4-8), strong energy bands were found between 460-690 Hz, 925-1845 Hz, 2075-2695 Hz, and a contiguous, less-intense band was present to 6300 Hz.

The energy produced by the Servox, Aurex, and Western Electric, when used by laryngectomees, appears to be somewhat modulated by the resonances of the vocal tract. The energy of the Barts, particularly between approximately 460 and 2000 Hz, is very intense and constant. Some formant movement can be seen superimposed on the broad band of energy. The undamped, aperiodic nature of this very intense band of energy is probably responsible for much of the unpleasant quality of the Barts and certainly affects intelligibility. Further, the amplitude modulations of the pulse beats of the Barts are 5 db when uncoupled and 3 db when coupled to tissue. The others are all 2.5 db and 2 db, respectively.

ACOUSTIC ANALYSIS OF SPEECH

Isshiki and Tanabe (1972) and Rothman (1978) have discussed characteristics of electronic artificial larynx speech, which serves to differentiate between superior, good, and poor talkers. The most distinguishing characteristic for the good and superior talkers includes the ability to produce differentiated voiced/ voiceless cognates for stop and fricative consonants with a consistently activated electronic larynx. This involves attenuating the larynx duty cycle and using buccal air. The differences between voiced and voiceless stop consonant closures as produced by superior electronic larynx talkers are not always appropriate; that is, they do not follow normal patterns. For example, voiced stop closures are often longer than those for voiceless closures in electronic larynx speech. However, a good electronic larynx talker would use the inappropriate longer closure duration time

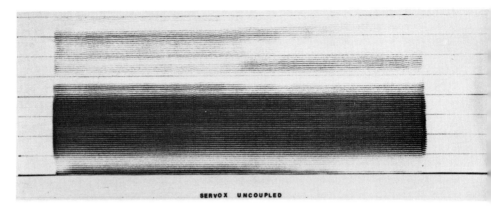

SERVOX UNCOUPLED

Figure 4-1. Narrow-band spectrogram of the output of the Servox uncoupled from tissue.

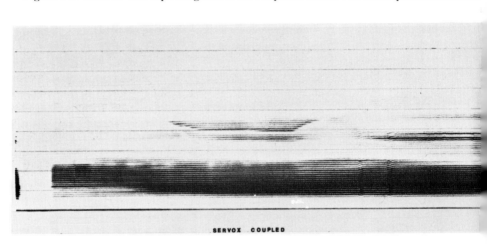

SERVOX COUPLED

Figure 4-2. Narrow-band spectrogram of the output of the Servox when coupled to tissue

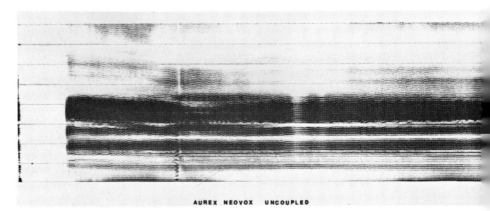

AUREX NEOVOX UNCOUPLED

Figure 4-3. Narrow-band spectrogram of the output of the Aurex Neovox uncouple from tissue.

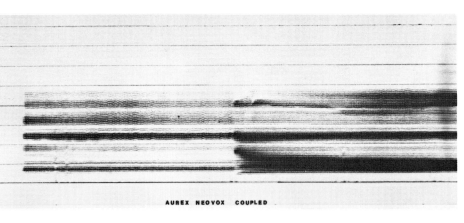

AUREX NEOVOX COUPLED

Figure 4-4. Narrow-band spectrogram of the output of the Aurex Neovox coupled to
tissue.

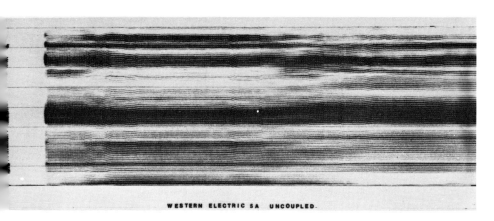

WESTERN ELECTRIC 5A UNCOUPLED

Figure 4-5. Narrow-band spectrogram of the output of the Western Electric 5A uncoupled
from tissue.

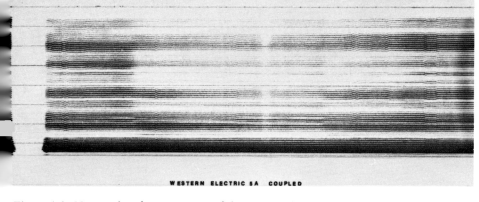

WESTERN ELECTRIC 5A COUPLED

Figure 4-6. Narrow-band spectrogram of the output of the Western Electric 5A coupled to
tissue.

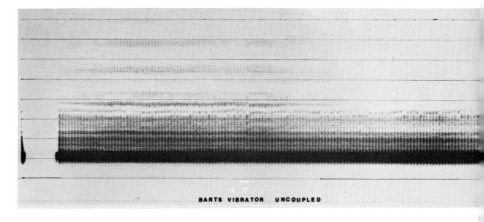

Figure 4-7. Narrow-band spectrogram of the output of the Barts Vibrator uncoupled fr(
tissue.

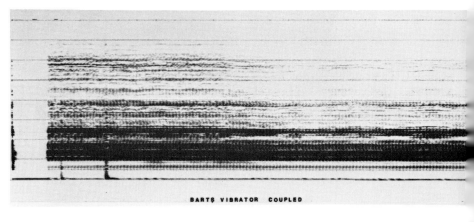

Figure 4-8. Narrow-band spectrogram of the output of the Barts Vibrator when cou[
to tissue.

to provide a voice bar (periodic energy), which is often a necessary component for distinguishing a voiced from voiceless stop. This can be seen in Figure 4-9—a wide-band spectrogram of a superior female talker using a Western Electric No. 5.

First, notice in Figure 4-9 how the vowel formants and transitions are appropriately modified by the changing resonance characteristics of the vocal tract. Notice, too, the segments

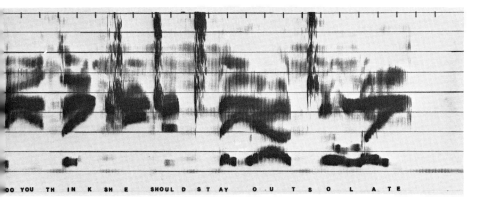

Figure 4-9. Wide-band spectrogram of superior female talker using a Western Electric 5A.
The orthographic representation of the sentence is spaced to approximate the appearance of
the associated acoustic events.

representing the /k/ of "think" and the /d/ of "should." The /k/
closure is shorter than that of /d/—60 msec for /k/ versus 85 msec
for /d/. However, the periodic pulse tone of the larynx is more
intense during the /d/ closure. The duty cycle of the larynx was
attenuated by 19 db between the vocalic /i/ and the /k/ and by
only 12 db between the vocalic /ʊ/ and the /d/. Strong frication
can be seen overlaid on the attenuated vibrations of the device
during productions of / ʃ / and /s/.

Figure 4-10 is an amplitude display of the same utterance.
Notice the broad peaks separated, for the most part, by rather
steep slopes indicating drops in intensity. This is a consistent
pattern distinguishing between good to superior and poor
electronic larynx users. In contrast, examine Figures 4-11 and 4-
12, which show a male talker reading the same sentence with a
Western Electric No. 5.

Examine the wide-band spectrogram of Figure 4-11. Notice the
predominance of energy bands throughout the spectrum. These
represent the output of the device undifferentiated by the vocal-
tract resonances. Also, notice the inappropriate pause between
"you" and "think." The talker shut the device down in order to
prepare for the voiceless /θ / in "think." Further, the closures for
the various voiced and voiceless stop consonants are poorly
distinguished. Attenuation during /k/ of "think" and /t/ of

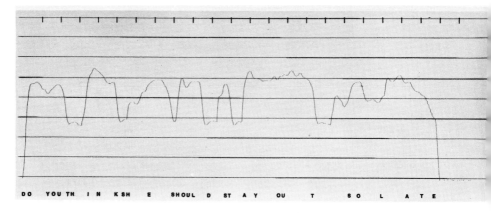

Figure 4-10. Averaged amplitude display generated from the production of the superior talker as illustrated in figure 4-9. The distance between each horizontal line represents 6 db.

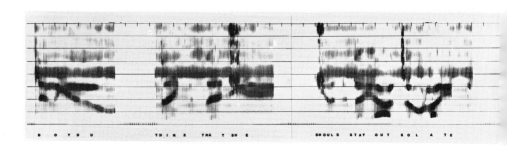

Figure 4-11. Wide-band spectrogram of a fair male talker using a Western Electric 5A. The orthographic representation of the sentence is spaced to approximate the appearance of the associated acoustic events.

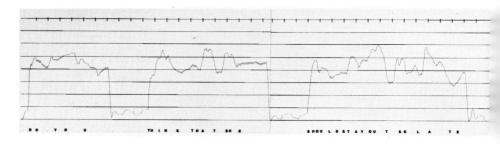

Figure 4-12. Averaged amplitude display generated from the production of the fair talker as illustrated in Figure 4-11. The distance between each horizontal line represents 6 db.

"that" is only between 10 and 13 db. Attenuation during /d/ of "should" is 14 db when measured from the vocalic /ʊ/ and only 5 db when measured from the /l/ portion. In the amplitude display of Figure 4-12, notice the constantly changing, random nature and poor differentiation of intensity changes. This talker has difficulty in differentiating consonantal elements and in maintaining appropriate consonant-vowel amplitude ratios.

Figures 4-13 and 4-14 show the wide-band spectrogram and amplitude display of the superior talker reading the second sentence of "The Rainbow Passage." Frequency range during the sentence varies from a high of 160 Hz to a low, at the end of the sentence, of 125 Hz. Inter-formant energy is absent or extremely attenuated as it would be in a spectrogram of a normal speaker. Fricatives are clearly distinguishable because high frequency artificial larynx energy is damped. Stop consonantal closures are clearly evident and are accompanied by an attenuation of the vibrator's pulse tone of at least 18 db. Further, this talker deactivated the vibrator before the final /s/ in "colors." It would be difficult to judge whether or not this spectrogram resulted from speech produced by a normal talker.

In contrast, Figures 4-15 and 4-16 represent speech produced by an average (i.e. fairly good) user of the Western Electric No. 5. Frequency variation is not used. The energy of the device is not being attenuated by the filter characteristics of the vocal tract. Attempts to attenuate the device for stop consonantal closure is evident in the amplitude display, but it is not as abrupt or as great as it is in the amplitude display of the superior talker. Further, the vocalic peaks are not as broad or clearly defined.

Without further controlled investigations, one can only speculate as to the differences observed in the spectrograms and amplitude displays of these two talkers (*see* Figures 4-13—4-16.) However, it is obvious that considerable attenuation of electronic larynx output will result when the vocal tract or the oral cavity aperture is closed as for stop consonants. Further, changing coupling pressure and pitch will cause changes in the radiated output of the device as it interacts with vocal-tract resonances. Figure 4-17 shows an uncoupled Western Electric's output vibrating at a rate of 150 Hz. Figures 4-18 and 4-19 show

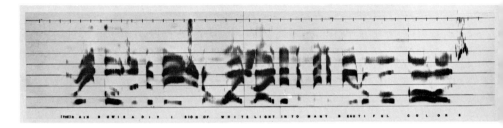

Figure 4-13. Wide-band spectrogram of a superior female talker using a Western Electric 5A. The orthographic representation of the sentence is spaced to approximate the appearance of the associated acoustic events.

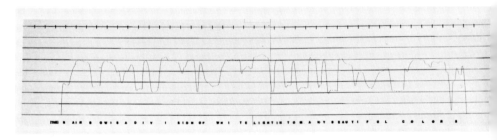

Figure 4-14. Averaged amplitude display generated from the production of the superior talker as illustrated in figure 4-12. The distance between each horizontal line represents 6 db.

the same device when coupled to the neck with medium and strong pressures, respectively.

Note the increase in the intensity of the energy between 3000-6000 Hz when coupling pressure is increased. Frequency is 170 Hz, and the vocal-tract configuration is such that the vowel /ɑ/ is being produced. Figures 4-20 and 4-21 show changes due to increasing pitch from 90-160 Hz when coupled to the neck with

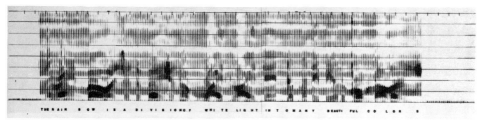

Figure 4-15. Wide-band spectrogram of a fair male talker using a Western Electric 5A. The orthographic representation of the sentence is spaced to approximate the appearance of the associated acoustic events.

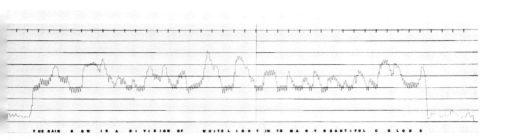

Figure 4-16. Averaged amplitude display generated from the production of the fair talker s illustrated in figure 4-15. The distance between each horizontal line represents 6 db.

medium pressure. Figure 4-22 shows the effect of stopping the vocal tract for the consonant /t/. Figures 4-18—4-22 were produced by an individual with a normal larynx, neck tissue, and associated musculature.

From the examples provided, it should be obvious that there is a large amount of variation in the use of the electronic larynx by different talkers. Further, development of a high level of speech

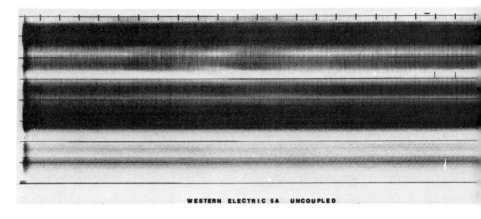

WESTERN ELECTRIC 5A   UNCOUPLED

Figure 4-17. Wide-band spectrogram of a Western Electric 5A uncoupled to tissue ar vibrating at a rate of 150 Hz.

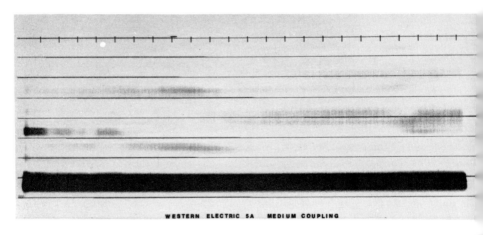

WESTERN ELECTRIC 5A   MEDIUM COUPLING

Figure 4-18. Wide-band spectrogram of a Western Electric 5A coupled to tissue wi medium pressure and vibrating at a rate of 170 Hz.

communication proficiency is possible with the electronic larynx. It is dependent on more than simple coupling to the tissues of the neck and learning to turn the device on and off. Use of pitch control, when available, with subtle variations in coupling pressure and use of buccal air can result in speech containing a multiplicity of cues necessary for adequate perception. Clinical use of the sound spectrograph can provide documentation for

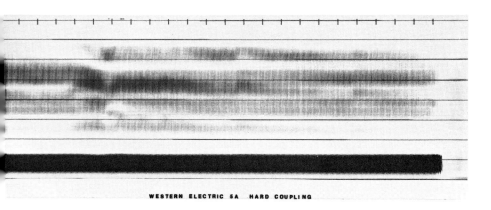

Figure 4-19. Wide-band spectrogram of a Western Electric 5A coupled to tissue with strong pressure and vibrating at a rate of 170 Hz.

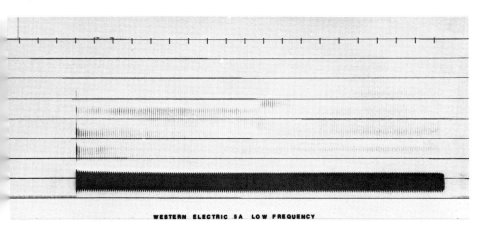

Figure 4-20. Wide-band spectrogram of a Western Electric 5A coupled to tissue with medium pressure and vibrating at a rate of 90 Hz.

differences in speech output. Videotape can be utilized to study thumb and hand movements of superior electronic larynx users as they vary and coordinate coupling pressure during the production of voiced and voiceless sounds. Strain gauges adapted to measure pressure or mechanical pressure transducers should be used so that changes in coupling pressure can be quantified and correlated with acoustic output.

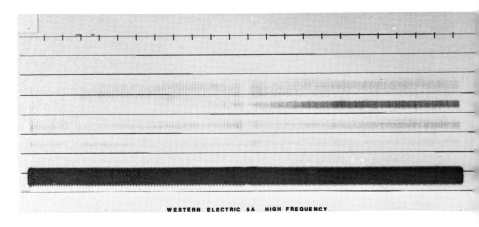

Figure 4-21. Wide-band spectrogram of a Western Electric 5A coupled to tissue wi
medium pressure and vibrating at a rate of 160 Hz.

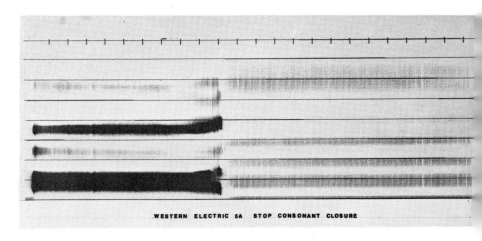

Figure 4-22. Wide-band spectrogram of a Western Electric 5A while the vocal trac
being stopped for the production of the consonant /t/.

SUMMARY

In summary, a high degree of speech communication proficiency can be achieved. Use of the electronic larynx must be
coordinated with articulation and manner of production. Coor-
dination of controls for activation/deactivation, pitch and differential coupling pressure for voicing onset and offset, and for

voiced and voiceless consonants must be controlled in a subtle manner in conjunction with the use of buccal air.

REFERENCES

Bennett, S., and Weinberg, B.: Acceptability ratings of normal esophageal and artificial larynx speech. *J Speech Hear Res, 61*:608-615, 1973.

Berry, W.R.: Attitudes of speech pathologists and otolaryngologists about artificial larynges. In *The Artificial Larynx Handbook.* New York: Grune, 1978.

Carter, J.: Personal communication. V.A. Hospital, Martinsburg, West Virginia, 1976.

Crouse, G.P.: "An Experimental Study of Esophageal and Artificial Larynx Speech." Unpublished M.S.Thesis, Emory University, 1962.

Goldstein, L.P.: Listener judgments of artificial larynx speech. In *The Artificial Larynx Handbook.* New York: Grune, 1978, chap. 4.

Goldstein, L.P.: "A study of the Relationship Between Adience-Abience Scale Scores and Judgements of Verbal Communication Proficiency of a Group of Esophageal Speakers and a Group of Artificial Larynx Speakers. Unpublished doctoral dissertation, University of Kansas, 1974.

Goldstein, L.P.: Review of the literature pertaining to the artificial larynx. *Proceedings of the Regional Medical Education Center,* Birmingham, Alabama: 1976.

Goldstein, L.P., and Rothman, H.: Analysis of artificial larynx speech: a preliminary report. *Proceedings of the Regional Medical Education Center,* Birmingham, Alabama: 1976.

Goode, R.: Artificial laryngeal devices in postlaryngectomy rehabilitation. *Laryngoscope, 135*:677-689, 1975.

Hyman, M.: An experimental study of artificial larynx and esophageal speech. *J Speech Hear Disord, 20*:291-299, 1955.

Isshiki, N., and Tanabe, M.: Acoustic and aerodynamic study of a superior electrolarynx speaker. *Folia Phoniatr, 24*:65-76, 1972.

Kallen, L.A.: Vicarious vocal mechanisms. *AMA Arch Otolaryngol, 20*:360-503, 1934.

Lauder, E.: The laryngectomee and the artificial larynx. *J Speech Hear Disord, 33*:147-157, 1968.

Lauder, E.: The laryngectomee and the artificial larynx—a second look. *J Speech Hear Disord, 35*:62-65, 1970.

Lauder, E.: *Self-Help for the Laryngectomee.* San Antonio, Texas, 1975.

Lebrun, Y.: *The Artificial Larynx,* Neurolinguistics series 1. Amsterdam: Swets and Zeitlinger, B.V., 1973.

McCroskey, R., and Mulligan, M.: The relative intelligibility of esophageal speech and artificial larynx speech. *J Speech Hear Disord, 28*: 37-41, 1963.

Morton, C.: *Modern Techniques of Vocal Rehabilitation.* Springfield, Thomas, 1973.

Rothman, H.B.: Analyzing artificial larynx speech. In *The Artificial Larynx Handbook*. New York: Grune, 1978.

Shames, G., Font, J., and Matthews, J.: Factors related to speech proficiency of the laryngectomized. *J Speech Hear Disord, 28*:273-287, 1963.

Stetson, R.H.: Can all laryngectomized patients be taught esophageal speech? *Trans American Laryngology Association, 59*:59-71, 1937.

ACOUSTIC AND PERCEPTUAL
FEATURES OF LARYNGEAL CANCER

THOMAS MURRY AND SADANAND SINGH

ABSTRACT

Vowel and phrase samples were recorded by five normal and five laryngeal pathology patients to measure physical and psychophysical factors and to subject them to a multidimensional analysis routine (ALSCAL). The physical measures obtained were f_0, F_1, F_2, airflow, and pitch perturbation factors. The psychophysical measures obtained were judgments of pitch, effort, breathiness, nasality, and roughness. The ALSCAL analysis of the similarity judgments of the paired, compared voice samples revealed a three-dimensional solution for both the vowel and phrase data. The judgments of vowel samples showed a much clearer separation of normal versus the laryngeal cancer patients than the judgments of the phrase samples. The physical and psychological measures were somewhat helpful in separating the laryngeal cancer and normal subjects. Some interesting interpretations of the solutions of ALSCAL factors are presented in terms of the obtained physical and psychophysical measures.

INTRODUCTION

THE CONFUSIONS THAT EXIST for normal voice categorization are magnified when classifying abnormal phonation. Roughness or "hoarseness" appears to be used for a multitude of laryngeal behaviors. These may range from psychologically based problems to disease-related conditions, such as growths on the vocal folds. Van Riper and Irwin (1958) describe hoarseness in terms of breathiness and harshness. Thurman (1953) reported that listeners often confused breathiness with hoarseness in perceptual test. Shipp and Huntington (1965) found a relationship between hoarseness and breathiness judgments for laryngitic patients, but they noted an inverse relationship between hoarse and harsh judgments.

Phonation is without a doubt a complex perceptual concept. Neither normal or abnormal phonation is accountable on any one perceptual dimension. Reports by Schmitke (1972), Murry and Schmitke (1975), Emanuel and Smith (1974), and Coleman (1971) all demonstrated that certain acoustic or physiologic parameters of normal or abnormal phonation have a perceptually related component such as roughness, hoarseness, or breathiness. For example, Schmitke measured mean air flow rate of 29 voices and then obtained judgments of breathiness. She found a 0.66 correlation between mean flow rate and perceived breathiness. Emanuel and Smith demonstrated a reduction in perceived vowel roughness as the speaking fundamental frequency was raised by one octave. Coleman found that an increase in roughness perception was related to an increase in the amplitude of the lower partials.

Since the concept of voice quality is complex, it is likely that listeners are responding to multiple cues from categorizing or differentiating voices. A method that allows for a posteriori determination of voice characteristics, known as INDSCAL, has been demonstrated as a feasible way of reducing perceptual confusions among voice qualities (Murry, Singh, and Sargent 1977). This empirical multidimensional analysis technique has previously been used to analyze a variety of stimuli with obscure or complex perceptual parameters. Shepard (1972), Mitchell and Singh (1974), and Danhauer and Singh (1975), to name just a few, have applied INDSCAL to the study of parameters utilized in phoneme perception. Murry, Singh, and Sargent (1977), Singh and Murry (1978), and Walden et al.(1978) have shown that INDSCAL can be applied to obtain the perceptual attributes associated with normal and abnormal voices. The Murry, Singh, and Sargent study data was obtained from a group of voices with various etiologies. The INDSCAL solution indicated that subjects clustered according to the presence or absence of a laryngeal mass lesion among other parameters. This clustering was related to a second formant feature. That is, those subjects with vocal-fold lesions showed relatively higher F2 than did those without a lesion. Since the types of lesions varied (benign versus malignant, bilateral versus unilateral, and radiated versus nonradiated), these data can only be considered as preliminary in terms of its diagnostic value. Moreover, the acoustic and physiologic parameters available to interpret these data showed some overlapping of the lesion versus nonlesion subjects.

This report is confined to a detailed analysis of subjects with laryngeal cancer and a normal group approximately the same age. The purpose of this study is to investigate the perceptual parameters of normal and abnormal male voices diagnosed as having laryngeal cancer. It is hypothesized that a finite number of perceptual cues for classifying voices are available from a listener's perceptual experience. These may include knowledge of physiological properties of the voice and speech mechanisms, in addition to acoustic and cultural traits often displayed in voices. In this study, acoustic and physiologic parameters were measured along with five psychophysical parameters. Similarity judgments of all possible voice pairs were obtained from fifteen listeners. These judgments were analyzed by a scaling procedure known as ALSCAL to determine what perceptual dimensions are available for categorizing the two divergent groups. ALSCAL presents a more robust treatment of the variance associated with individuals than does INDSCAL. In addition, the data may be in rank order rather than numerical. ALSCAL makes no assumptions about the quality of any two items in a given comparison. For this study, similarity judgments of all stimuli presented in pairs provided the input to ALSCAL.

PROCEDURE

Subjects

Ten subjects included five with no observable laryngeal disorder and five diagnosed as having laryngeal cancer. The patients with laryngeal cancer ranged in age from 61 - 69 years, with a mean age of 65.2 years. Their voice samples were obtained after biopsy confirmation of malignant tissue and prior to total laryngectomy surgery. All five subsequently underwent wide-field total laryngectomy surgery. Based on the current medical nomenclature (American Joint Committee 1977) for describing the tumor condition, three subjects had $T_2 N_1 M_0$ lesions, and two subjects had $T_3 N_1 M_0$ lesions. The primary site of lesion for each subject was the true vocal folds, and, for all cases, indirect laryngoscopic examination revealed vocal-fold movement. No one was selected for this study if the tumor resulted in fixation of the vocal folds or if the vocal output appeared to preclude acoustic analysis of the periodic components. The subjects might be considered to represent a group with moderate vocal roughness; none spoke in a whisper or aphonia.

The normal subjects ranged from 55 - 71 years, with a mean age of 63.8 years. All denied any history of voice problems, and all were in apparent good health. Indirect laryngoscopic examinations performed on the normal subjects verified the normal status of the vocal folds; no abnormalities were observed.

Method

One speech sample used for the analysis consisted of the sustained vowel $/a/$. The subjects were instructed to produce the vowel in a comfortable manner for at least two seconds. Each subject stood in a double-walled, sound-treated room 25 centimeters away from an Electrovoice® 654 microphone. The microphone output was directed to a Revox® A-77 magnetic tape recorder playing at 7.5 ips.

The subjects also read a standard passage (Fairbanks 1960). From the third sentence of this *"Rainbow Passage,"* the mean fundamental frequency was obtained through Visicorder analysis. The magnetic tapes were low-pass filtered at 500 Hz before producing the oscillographic record. To compute the mean fundamental frequency (f_0), the number of waveforms occurring in each 0.1 second segment were counted. An f_0 based on one sentence was computed by multiplying the values for each segment by 10 and dividing by the total number of phonated segments.

To obtain the perturbation measures from the sustained vowel, a technique described by Hollien, Michel, and Doherty (1973) was employed. The method was shown to be valid when used to measure synthetic signals with predetermined perturbation characteristics. Basically, a continuous unframed film was made of the speech signal, along with a 5.0 kHz square-wave reference tone, using a Fastax® camera. After the film was developed, the consecutive periods of the voice signal were marked and timed to the nearest 0.1 msec. The values then were averaged to obtain the mean perturbation for the vowel. The complete and fractional reference cycles within one glottal waveform were summed and the period of waveform in question was calculated using the formula:

$$\frac{\text{Nrs}}{\text{Frs}} = \text{Pvs, where}$$

Nrs = The number of reference signal cycles
Frs = The frequency of the reference signal in kilohertz
Pvs = The period of the vocal signal in milliseconds

Two observers working independently provided all the Pvs measures. If the two observers differed by more than 0.1 msec, the entire set of reference cycles for the period were remeasured. The data were converted to frequency and normalized for differences in mean f_0 for the formula:

$$\text{Jitter Factor (JF)} = \frac{\text{mean Jitter} \times 100}{\text{mean } f_0}$$

The jitter factor reported in percent of the mean f_0 for sustained phonation is comparable to the measure of frequency magnitude perturbation factor (MPF) for conversation speech described by Lieberman (1961).

The directional perturbation factor (DPF) was obtained by tabulating the number of periodic waveform directional changes in the entire signal relative to the total number of waveforms in the signal.

Psychophysical Analysis

The vowel /ɑ/ and the phrase, "These take the shape of a long round arch," were reproduced ten times in random order on a test tape. All samples were recorded on a master tape at a constant VU level to assure equal loudness upon playback.

Similarity Judgments

Fifteen subjects—students and department members of a speech pathology clinic—served as the listeners. Each listener was asked to rate the voice on a seven-point scale for one of five qualities: pitch, effort, breathiness, nasality, and roughness. All listeners in this group were familiar with voice-rating scales and all had experience with voice-disordered patients.

Data Analysis

The following acoustic and physiologic parameters were measured. For the vowel: mean f_o, airflow rate, F_1, F_2, F_2-F_1, F_2/F_1, MPF, and DPF were obtained. For the phrase: f_o mean and f_o standard deviation, mean F_1, F_2, F_2-F_1, and F_2/F_1 for all vowels, vocalic duration within the phrase, duration of the phrase, and the ratio of vocalic duration to total duration were the measures used to interpret the ALSCAL solution. In addition, five perceptual measures (pitch, effort, breathiness, nasality, and roughness) were obtained for the vowel and the phrase.

RESULTS

Physical Measures

Tables 5-I and 5-III show the acoustic/physiological data for the vowel and the phrase, respectively. The data for each measure are presented in rank order from the highest to the lowest. In all instances, subjects 1-5 are the normal subjects and 6-10 are those with laryngeal cancer. The mean values of each measure, along with the mean rank for each group, and the difference in the mean ranks between the two groups are shown at the bottom of each table. C represents the mean for the cancer patients and N for the normals. The final three pairs of columns in Table 5-I refers to the perturbation measures obtained from the subjects and the airflow rates. The final three pairs of columns in Table 5-III refers to durational measures of the phrase.

Table 5-I. Rank Order and Subject Number for the Acoustic and Physiologic Measures of the Vowel Stimuli. The Mean Values and Mean Ranks are Shown at the Bottom.

Rank	X̄f₀	s	F₁	s	F₂	s	F₂-F₁	s	F₂/F₁	s	MPF (%)	s	DPF (%)	s	X̄ Air-Flow	s
1	215.7	9	999.0	8	1352.5	8	610.5	1	2.00	6	7.91	9	65.3	8	420.5	6
2	132.0	5	849.4	4	1276.5	5	580.5	5	1.94	1	2.33	7	65.3	5	418.0	9
3	127.9	2	832.5	3	1258.0	1	573.5	6	1.83	5	1.80	10	63.3	1	251.5	10
4	126.7	4	795.5	2	1202.5	9	499.5	7	1.73	7	1.49	2	61.2	6	175.0	8
5	123.9	3	740.0	9	1184.0	7	462.5	9	1.63	9	1.27	8	61.1	2	166.0	1
6	115.8	10	728.9	10	1170.3	4	381.1	10	1.52	10	1.09	5	60.0	10	109.5	2
7	111.9	7	696.0	5	1147.0	6	363.5	8	1.38	4	0.82	1	59.2	9	83.0	7
8	111.4	6	684.5	7	1110.0	3	320.9	4	1.35	2	0.79	4	57.1	3	73.5	5
9	110.0	1	647.5	1	1110.0	10	277.5	2	1.35	8	0.77	6	55.1	7	72.0	4
10	85.7	8	573.5	6	1073.0	2	277.5	3	1.33	3	0.76	3	45.8	4	64.0	3
X̄ C	131.3		745.2		1199.2		454.0		1.65		2.82		60.2		269.9	
N	120.9		784.2		1177.6		413.4		1.57		0.99		58.5		97.0	
X̄ Rank C	5.6		6.0		5.2		5.0		4.90		4.00		5.5		3.4	
N	5.4		5.0		5.8		6.0		6.10		7.00		5.5		7.6	
Difference	0.2		1.0		0.8		1.0		1.20		3.00		0.0		4.2	

Psychophysical Measures

Tables 5-II and 5-IV present the ranked psychophysical ratings for each subject for the vowel and phrase, respectively. The overall mean rating for the two subgroups, the mean rank, and the differences between the mean ranks are shown at the bottom of the tables. The data from these four tables were the basis for interpretation of the ALSCAL solutions for the vowel and phrase.

Multidimensional Analysis (ALSCAL)

For the vowel, a three-dimensional ALSCAL solution was the most appropriate. Figure 5-1 is a plot of dimension 1 and 2 of the 3-D solution. The dashed line in this figure is primarily for visual separation of dimension 2 (D2). Dimension 1 (D1) appears to be a categorical dimension in that it separates the normal subjects (1, 2, 3, 4, 5) from those with laryngeal cancer (6, 7, 8, 9, 10). D1 may also be interpreted in terms of mean airflow rate, breathiness, effort, and roughness. In all four instances, subjects with a high

Table 5-II. Rank Order and Subject Number for each of Five Psychophysical Ratings of the Vowel Stimuli. All Ratings are Based on a Seven Point Scale.

Rank	Pitch	S	Effort	S	Breathiness	S	Nasality	S	Roughness	S
1	4.71	5	6.79	9	6.50	9	4.25	8	6.43	10
2	4.64	4	6.32	10	5.89	10	3.89	4	5.71	6
3	4.32	9	5.18	6	5.61	6	3.46	5	5.54	7
4	4.21	3	5.00	7	4.00	7	3.00	1	5.39	9
5	3.29	2	3.89	8	3.57	8	2.75	7	5.14	8
6	3.25	1	3.32	4	2.46	4	2.68	2	3.64	4
7	2.82	7	3.14	5	2.39	5	2.39	10	3.07	2
8	2.18	10	2.93	2	2.25	2	2.57	3	2.93	5
9	1.79	6	2.14	3	2.00	3	2.46	6	2.43	3
10	1.57	8	1.93	1	1.61	1	1.46	9	2.21	1
$\overline{X}$ C	2.54		5.44		5.11		2.72		5.64	
N	4.02		2.69		2.14		3.12		2.86	
$\overline{X}$ Rank C	7.40		3.00		3.00		6.30		3.00	
N	3.60		8.00		8.00		4.70		8.00	
Difference	3.80		5.00		5.00		1.60		5.00	

Table 5-III. Rank Order and Subject Number for Each of the Nine Acoustic and Temporal Measures of the Phrase Stimuli. The Frequency Measures in the Six Pairs of Columns are in Hertz. All Duration Measures are in Seconds.

Rank	$\overline{X}f_0$	S	SDf_0	S	$\overline{X}F_1$	S	$\overline{X}F_2$	S	F_2-F_1	S	F_2/F_1	S	Phrase Duration	S	Vocalic Duration	S	Voc/phrase Duration	S
1	176.4	9	21.3	10	730.4	9	2183.2	10	1463.2	10	3.03	10	3.57	8	3.34	6	0.93	1
2	137.7	4	20.4	9	720.0	10	1920.0	9	1189.6	9	2.70	7	3.73	6	2.93	10	0.93	3
3	130.6	5	18.5	8	575.5	8	1493.0	7	939.5	7	2.69	5	3.34	10	2.90	8	0.92	5
4	128.7	3	16.8	2	572.0	6	1472.0	6	900.0	6	2.68	4	3.00	5	2.77	5	0.92	9
5	125.8	10	14.4	5	553.5	7	1382.4	4	866.8	4	2.63	9	2.95	9	2.71	9	0.90	6
6	121.3	7	13.1	6	515.6	4	1375.6	5	864.4	5	2.57	6	2.90	2	2.57	1	0.89	2
7	113.1	1	11.9	1	511.2	1	1369.0	8	793.5	8	2.38	8	2.77	1	2.57	2	0.89	7
8	106.7	8	11.3	3	449.6	3	1011.0	1	581.1	1	2.37	1	2.75	7	2.46	7	0.88	10
9	104.0	2	9.9	7	425.9	7	969.0	2	521.8	2	2.23	3	2.48	4	2.19	3	0.87	4
10	103.9	4	6.0	4	422.6	4	944.4	3	519.4	3	2.16	2	2.35	3	2.15	4	0.81	8
$\overline{X}$ C	126.8		16.6		630.3		1687.4		1057.2		2.66		3.27		2.87		0.88	
N	122.8		12.1		465.0		1136.5		670.7		2.43		2.70		2.45		0.91	
$\overline{X}$ Rank C	6.0		4.2		3.0		3.4		3.4		4.20		3.80		3.80		6.60	
N	5.0		6.8		8.0		7.6		7.6		6.80		7.20		7.20		4.40	
Difference	1.0		2.6		5.0		4.2		4.2		2.60		3.40		3.40		2.20	

Table 5-IV. Rank Order and Subject Number for Each of Five Psychophysical Ratings of the Phrase Stimuli. All Ratings are Based on a Seven-point Scale.

Rank	Pitch	S	Effort	S	Breathiness	S	Nasality	S	Roughness	S
1	4.32	9	6.71	10	6.82	9	5.54	8	6.46	10
2	4.18	3	6.29	9	6.82	10	2.89	2	5.79	6
3	4.14	5	5.36	6	5.29	6	3.71	7	5.57	7
4	4.04	10	4.54	7	3.93	7	3.57	1	5.39	9
5	3.86	4	3.14	4	3.18	8	3.50	5	3.29	8
6	3.46	1	2.61	5	2.61	4	3.46	3	3.21	4
7	3.39	8	2.57	8	2.07	5	3.25	4	2.79	2
8	3.32	2	2.54	2	1.79	1	3.25	6	2.61	1
9	2.43	7	2.25	1	1.79	2	2.04	9	2.21	5
10	1.96	6	2.04	3	1.75	3	2.04	10	2.07	3
$\overline{X}$ C	3.23		5.09		5.21		3.32		5.30	
N	3.79		2.52		2.00		3.33		2.58	
$\overline{X}$ Rank C	6.20		3.40		3.00		6.10		3.00	
$\overline{X}$ Rank N	4.80		7.60		8.00		4.90		8.00	
Difference	1.40		4.20		5.00		1.20		5.00	

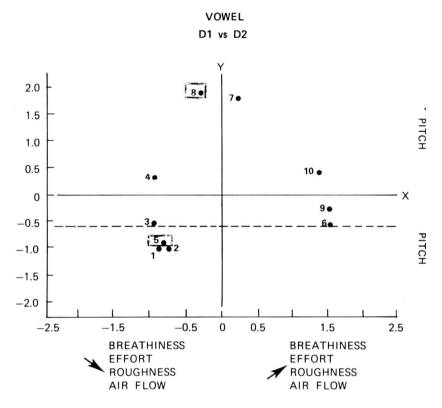

Figure 5-1. Plot of Dimension 1 and Dimension 2 of a three-dimensional vowel sample solution. D1 separates normal from laryngeal-cancer patients.

mean airflow rate or a high perceptual ranking on breathiness, effort, and roughness clustered on the right side, while those with a low mean airflow rate and scale value for the three psychophysical judgments were grouped on the left for this dimension. D1 clearly reflects a complex physio-perceptual dimension.

D2 can best be interpreted as a pitch dimension with the exceptions of S's 5 and 8, which were misclassified. Misclassification is illustrated as a box. Those subjects above the broken line were generally perceived as having higher pitch than those below the line.

Figure 5-2 is a plot of D1 versus D3. Using the data in Tables 5-I and 5-II the third dimension appears to be primarily an f_0

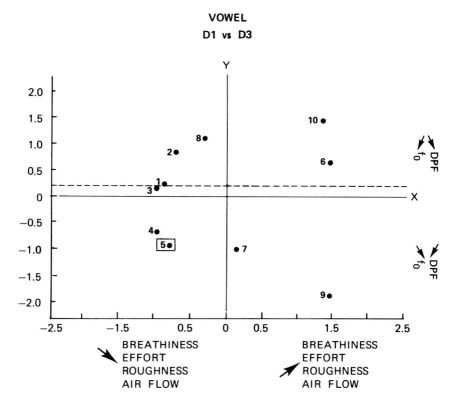

Figure 5-2. Plot of Dimension 1 and Dimension 3 of a three-dimensional vowel sample solution. D1, again, separates laryngeal-cancer and normal patients.

dimension. Subjects 6, 8, 10, 1, 2, and 3 have lower f_0 values than do subjects 7, 9, 4, and 5. Further examination of Figure 5-2 indicates that the directional perturbation factor (DPF) contributes to this solution also with the misclassification of subject number 5. To summarize the vowel data (D1), the physio-perceptual dimension categorically separates the normal subjects from those with laryngeal cancer.

Figures 5-3 and 5-4 present the scatter plots of D1/D2 and D1/D3 for the phrase. Again, D1 may be explained in terms of normal versus cancer with the exception of subject 8—a cancer subject who is clustered with the normals. The coordinates for

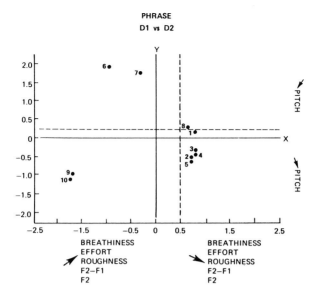

Figure 5-3. Plot of Dimension 1 and Dimension 2 of a three-dimensional phrase sample solution. D1 separates (with Subject 8 as an exception) laryngeal-cancer patients from the normals. D2 reflects the utilization of f_0 in speech perception.

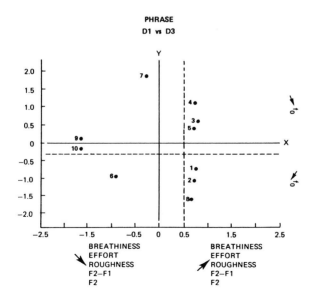

Figure 5-4. Plot of Dimension 1 and Dimension 3 of a three-dimensional phrase sample solution. D1, again, is mainly a cancer/normal division. D3 reflects the utilization of f_0 in voice perception.

subject 8 as well as ranked data of Tables 5-III and 5-IV suggest that subject 8 had vocal qualities more like the five normal subjects than the other four cancer subjects. The other four pathological subjects are clustered to the left. It is interesting to note the size of the two clusters. For the normals, the cluster is tightly grouped, while for the four cancer subjects there is a greater variability—a commonly accepted characteristic of pathological voices.

D1 also may be explained on the basis of two acoustic features, F2 and F2-F1, and the three perceptual features of roughness, breathiness, and effort.

D2 for the phrase sample is a pitch dimension, with the exception of subject 2, who was perceived as having low pitch but classified by ALSCAL in the high-pitch cluster.

D3 shown in Figure 5-4 may be interpreted as an f_0 dimension, with subjects 1, 2, 6, and 8 having low f_0 and the remaining subjects in the high f_0 group.

The phrase data may then be summarized as containing a vocal-tract perceptual dimension, similar to the physio-perceptual dimension of the vowels, a pitch dimension, and a frequency or laryngeal dimension. None of the three dimensions separated the normal and cancer groups categorically.

The data from the present study indicate that the perceptual attributes of normal and pathological voices appear to be a function of laryngeal and vocal-tract parameters. The acoustic laryngeal feature of f_0 was not sufficient to separate normal from pathologic. However, the physiologic measures of mean airflow rate did divide the subjects appropriately. The perceptual correlate of airflow rate, namely, perceived breathiness, was a distinguishing feature of the vowel and phrase stimuli.

Table 5-V shows the percentage of variance accounted for by each of the dimensions. The total variance accounted for by the three-dimension solution for the vowel was 69.8 percent; for the phrase, it was 76.2 percent of the total percentages. D1, the complex physio-perceptual dimension, accounted for 52.9 percent of the variance for the vowel condition and 61.9 percent of the variance for the phrase. Obviously, the higher amount of accounted variance for the phrase sample may be due to the

Table 5-V. Percentage of Variance Accounted for by Each of
the Three INDSCAL Dimensions for the Vowel and Phrase Conditions

Dimension	Percentage of variance accounted for	
	Vowel	Phrase
1	52.9	61.9
2	11.3	9.6
3	5.6	4.7
Total	69.8	76.2

greater amount of information regarding vocal function available to the listeners in the phrase sample than in the vowel sample.

SUMMARY

The present study supports the notion that perceptual categorization of voices is done using laryngeal and vocal-tract information. The physiologic measures of airflow, the acoustic measures of f_o, F_2 and F_2-F_1, and the perceptual features of pitch, breathiness, effort, and roughness all contribute to separate normal subjects from those with laryngeal cancer.

In previous studies of normal phonation, phrase data was considered to contribute to listener's ability to categorize voices. Since phrase data are costly to analyze, it is encouraging to find that analysis of the vowel data in the present study adequately separates the normal from the pathological subjects.

It is of interest to note that in a previous study of pathological voices (Murry, Singh, and Sargent 1977), five dimensions were required to interpret a solution from stimuli produced by subjects with a variety of dysphonias. In this study, the only pathology was laryngeal cancer, and three dimensions provided the best solution. Further application of ALSCAL to the study of vocal features for both normal and pathological conditions appears to be warranted based on the results of this study.

REFERENCES

American Joint Commission for Cover Staging and End Results Reports. *Manual for Staging of Cancer 1977*, American Cancer Society, New York, 1977.

Coleman, R.F.: Effect of waveform changes upon roughness perception. *Folia Phoniatr, 23*:314-322, 1971.

Danhauer, J.L. and Singh, S.: *Multidimensional Speech Perception by Hearing Impaired.* Baltimore: Univ. Park, 1975.

Fairbanks, G.: *Voice and Articulation Drillwork.* New York: Har-Row, 1960.

Emanual, F., and Smith, W.: Pitch effects on vowel roughness and spectral noise. *J Phonetics, 2*:247-253, 1974.

Hollien, H., Michel, J., and Doherty, E.T.: A method for analyzing vocal jitter in sustained phonation. *J Phonetics, 1*:85-91, 1973.

Lieberman, P.: Perturbations in vocal pitch. *J Acoust Soc Am., 33*:597-602, 1961.

Mitchell, L. and Singh, S.: Perceptual structure of sixteen prevocalic English consonants sententially embedded. *J Acoust Soc Am, 55*:1355-1357, 1974.

Murry, T. and Schmitke, L.: Airflow onset and variability. *Folia Phoniatr, 27*: 401-409, 1975.

Murry, T., Singh, S., and Sargent, M.: Multidimensional classification of abnormal voice qualities. *J Acoust Soc Am, 61*:1630-1635, 1977.

Schmitke, L.: "Correlation of Airflow Measurements with Degrees of Perceived Breathiness." M.A. thesis, San Diego State University, 1972.

Shepard, R.N.: Psychological representation of speech sounds. In David, E.E. Jr., and Denes, P.B.: *A Unified View.* New York: McGraw-Hill, 1972.

Shipp, T. and Huntington, D.: Some acoustic and perceptual factors in acute-laryngitic hoarseness. *J Speech Hear Disord, 30*:350-359, 1965.

Singh, S. and Murry, T.: Multidimensional classification of normal voice qualities. *J Acoust Soc Am, 64*:81-87, 1978.

Thurman, W.L.: "The Constructed and Acoustic Analysis of Recorded Scales of Severity for Six Voice Quality Disorders." Ph.D. dissertation, Purdue University, 1953.

Van Riper, C. and Irwin, J. V.: *Voice and Articulation.* Englewood Cliffs,: P-H, 1958.

Walden, B.E., Montgomery, A., Gibeily, G., Prosek, R., and Schwartz, D.: Correlates of psychological dimensions in talker similarity. *J Speech Hear Research, 21*: 265-275, 1978.

PART II:
ELECTROACOUSTIC
SPEECH AIDS

Chapter 6

HISTORY AND DEVELOPMENT OF LARYNGEAL PROSTHETIC DEVICES

LEWIS P. GOLDSTEIN

ABSTRACT

Concurrent with the first successful laryngectomy in 1873, the first successful prosthetic device for speech was developed. Josef Leiter was probably the first to devise an internal pneumatic laryngeal prosthesis. Over the next 100 years the principles and designs of these devices changed as medicine and technology advanced. The most significant change that broadened and expanded the development of laryngeal prosthetic devices occurred with the introduction of the first electrolarynx in 1940. Today the laryngectomized individual is able to choose from a variety of internal and external pneumatic or electronic laryngeal-prosthetic devices. Along with the historical development, various opinions and comparisons of the devices will be explored.

A N ARTIFICIAL LARYNX is a device used to simulate an approximation to normal laryngeal tones. They have been developed mainly for individuals who have had their larynx surgically removed. The quality of sound, the ease of use, and other physical attributes varies greatly for each device. It is impossible to say whether one device is better than another, since the individual's ability to use a device, the extent of surgery, and the amount of training as well as many other variables will make the output of the same device different for each patient.

There are many types of devices, and they all fall into two broad areas, as determined by the energy source (*see* Fig. 6-1). Therefore, we have devices that are either *electronic* or *pneumatic*. Each of

137

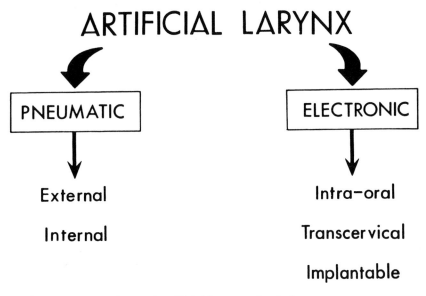

Figure 6-1. Breakdown of artificial larynges by their energy source.

these can be broken down into subclasses. A pneumatic prosthesis can be either *internal* or *external*. The electronic prosthesis can be *intraoral, transcervical or implantable*. Since the external pneumatic artificial larynx was the first to be developed, it will also serve as the beginning of our discussion.

External Pneumatic Devices

The first external pneumatic device was developed by Johann Czermack in 1854. The device was designed for an eighteen-year-old girl, who was tracheotomized because of complete laryngeal stenosis. The device consisted of a tube from the tracheostoma to the mouth. Inserted in the tube was a small metal reed that produced a sound as the air passed through it. The quality was poor, with the patient only producing single syllables.

A major criticism of Czermack's device was that the sound was delivered into the mouth rather than to the pharynx. In 1892, Hockenegg developed a device that consisted of a bellows, for air supply, connecting with a tube that was inserted through the nose into the pharynx. Midway into the tube was a reed for sound production (*see* Fig. 6-2).

The next external pneumatic artificial larynx was designed by George Gottstein in 1899 (*see* Fig. 6-3). His device consisted of a tracheal cannula, rubber tubing, a reed, a valve for air intake, and a mouthpiece. Attempts were made to have the device cosmetically pleasing and to hide the tubing within the patient's beard. However, with a short tube from the tracheostoma to the mouth, the individual could not move his head.

In the early 1920s, John Mackenty, an otolaryngologist, along with Harvey Fletcher and Charles Lane, engineers from Western Electric Company, developed an artificial larynx with a soft-rubber tracheal pad and tube that could be strapped over the tracheostoma, a cylinder containing a rubber band that could be adjusted for pitch, and a mouthpiece. The cylinder contained a hole for inhalation, and with digital closure, sound would be produced.

The Western Electric No. 1 was redesigned and replaced by the Western Electric No. 2 (*see* Fig. 6-4). The major difference was a slightly curved bronze reed replacing the rubber band enabling the device to be smaller and need less care. There was no need for periodically changing and tightening the rubber band.

The devices described thus far are collectors' items. Those external pneumatic devices that are currently available include:

1. The Van Humen (DSP8) artificial larynx (*see* Fig. 6-5). It consists of an adjustable rubber membrane with a nylon housing; an air-filled cuff fits over the stoma.
2. The Osaka artificial larynx (*see* Fig. 6-6) also uses a rubber membrane for sound production. The pitch and loudness can be altered by physically changing the membrane and by varying the breath pressure during speech.
3. The Neher 5000 (*see* Fig. 6-7) consists of a hard-plastic reed that can be altered in length, width, and shape to vary the pitch and tone initiation characteristics.
4. The Tokyo artificial larynx (*see* Fig. 6-8) can be obtained with either a steel or soft-rubber cover that fits over the stoma. This is attached to a chamber that houses a rubber membrane and terminates with a plastic or rubber mouth-

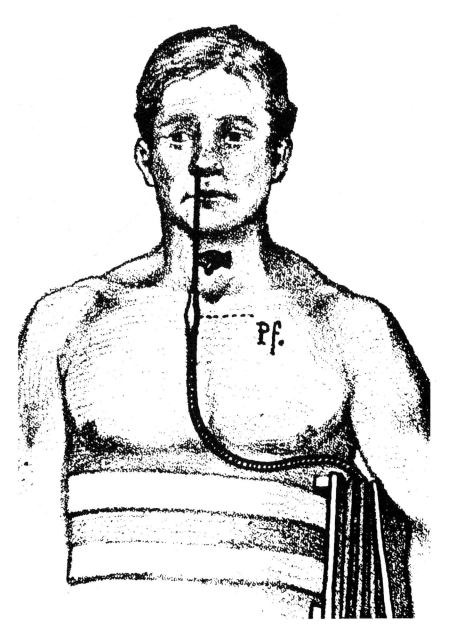

Figure 6-2. Artificial larynx developed by Hockenegg 1892. (Reprinted with permission. *The Artificial Larynx*, Yvan Lebrun. Swets and Zeitlinger, B.V. Amsterdam 1973.)

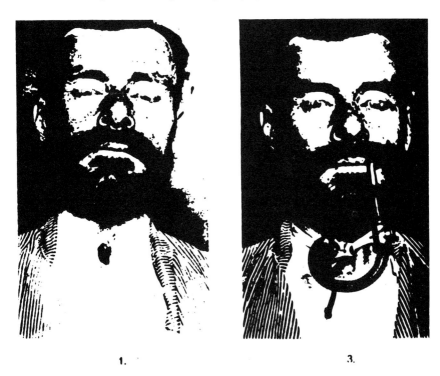

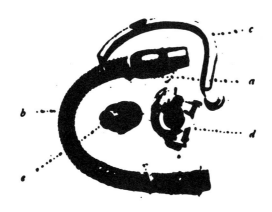

Figure 6-3. Artificial larynx developed by Gottstein 1899. (Reprinted with permission. *The Artificial Larynx*. Yvan Lebrun. Swets and Zeitlinger, B.V. Amsterdam 1973.)

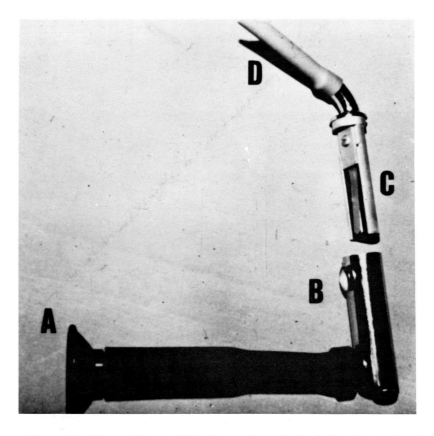

Figure 6-4. Western Electric #2. A. Stoma Cover. B. Reed Chamber. C. Reed. D. Mouth-tube. (Reprinted with permission. *The Artificial Larynx Handbook.* Salmon and Goldstein, eds. Grune and Stratton, N.Y. 1978.)

tube. This device has received a few modifications (Nelsen, Parkin, and Potter 1975). These include:

   a. Finger—control breath port (*see* Fig. 6-9)

   b. Rigid and curved mouth tubing (*see* Fig. 6-9)

   c. Swivel joint connector for stoma cover (*see* Fig. 6-10)

5. Since there has been renewed interest in the external pneumatic artificial larynx, the Western Electric No. 2 device has been considered for remanufacture; however, to date it is still not available.

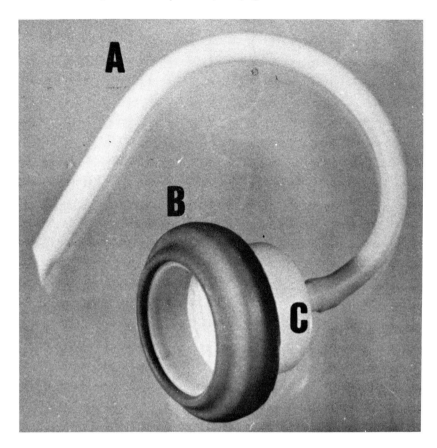

Figure 6-5. VanHumen (DSP8) Artificial Larynx. A. Mouth-tube. B. Vibratory mechanism. C. Stoma cover. (Reprinted with permission. *The Artificial Larynx Handbook.* Salmon and Goldstein, eds. Grune and Stratton, N.Y. 1978.)

Internal Pneumatic Devices

The first internal pneumatic artificial larynx was developed as a result of the first successful laryngectomy. Dr. Billroth, in 1873, removed the larynx but left a passage between the windpipe and the pharynx. Joseph Leiter devised a prosthesis that was inserted between the trachea and the pharynx; it was comprised of three cannulas: a tracheal, a laryngeal, and a phonatory cannula with a

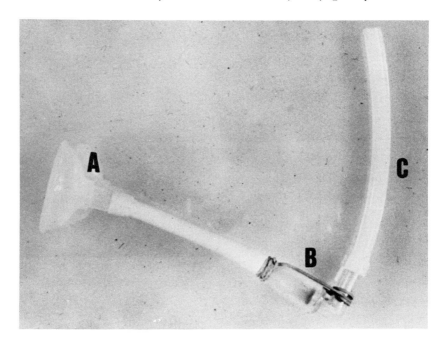

Figure 6-6. Osaka Artificial Larynx. A. Stoma cover. B. Vibratory mechanism. C. Mouth-tube. (Reprinted with permission, *The Artificial Larynx Handbook*. Salmon and Goldstein, eds. Grune and Stratton, N.Y. 1978.)

metal reed. The upper end of the laryngeal cannula had a lid held open by a spring that was to act like an epiglottis (*see* Fig. 6-11). In order to talk, the patient held a finger over the tracheostoma.

In 1874, Carl Gussenbauer improved Leiter's prosthesis by moving the reed closer to the tracheostoma so it could be easily removed and cleaned, since the artificial epiglottis was not very efficient. The reed remained metal, and the addition of a respirator helped filter the air that was inhaled (*see* Fig. 6-12).

Julius Wolf, in 1893, set out to remedy many of the flaws of the artificial larynx. He shortened the laryngeal cannula and lengthened the phonatory cannula, thus allowing the reed to be increased in size and placed higher. A fine-mesh sieve was placed over the phonatory cannula; this eliminated saliva from entering the device during speech. Further, a cork was used to plug the phonatory cannula during eating. Figure 6-13 pictures this

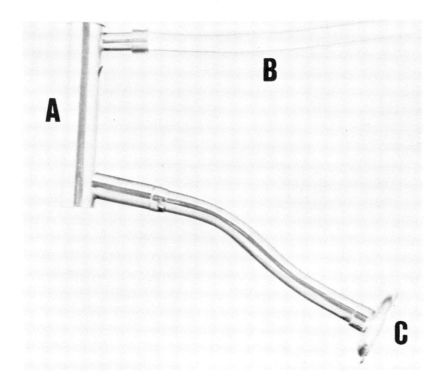

Figure 6-7. Neher 5000 Artificial Larynx. A. Reed. B. Mouth-tube. C. Stoma cover. (Reprinted with permission. *The Artificial Larnyx Handbook,* Salmon and Goldstein, eds. Grune and Stratton, N.Y. 1978.)

device, and a schematic of the device is seen in Figure 6-14. (It was reported that the patient could speak distinctly and also sing.)

In the early 1900s, surgical techniques changed. The passage-way between the pharynx and trachea was no longer routinely made. This led to designs of prostheses that were external. Recently there has been interest in surgical reconstruction for voice restoration. Emphasis has been on both, with and without the incorporation of a prosthesis.

In 1972, Taub reported a combination of a surgical and prosthetic approach to voice restoration. A fistula is formed surgically between the esophagus and skin surface. After healing, an external air-bypass prosthesis is inserted between the tracheo-stoma and the newly created fistula. Voice is produced by a

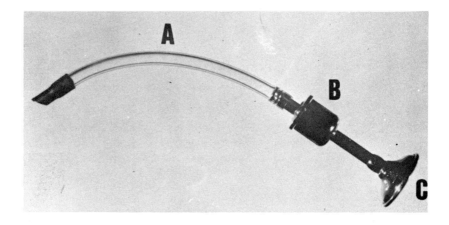

Figure 6-8. Tokyo Artificial Larynx. A. Mouth-tube. B. Vibratory mechanism. C. Stoma cover. (Reprinted with permission. *The Artificial Larynx Handbook.* Salmon and Goldstein, eds. Grune and Stratton, N.Y. 1978.)

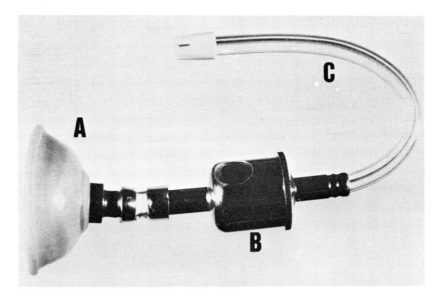

Figure 6-9. Tokyo artificial larynx with A. Soft rubber cover. B. Finger-control breath port. C. Rigid mouth tubing. (Reprinted with permission. *The Artificial Larynx Handbook.* Salmon and Goldstein, eds. Grune and Stratton, N.Y. 1978.)

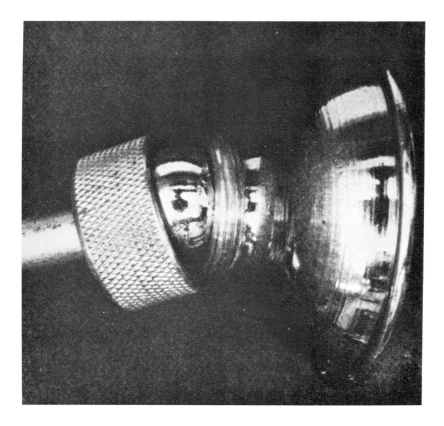

Figure 6-10. Swivel joint connector for the Tokyo artificial larynx. (Reprinted with permission. *Archives of Otolaryngology, 101*:108, 1975. Copyright 1975, American Medical Association.)

vibrating esophagus powered by the pulmonary air (*see* Fig. 6-15).

Shedd and his colleagues (1972) have developed a reed-fistula method of voice restoration. This method requires a surgically created fistula leading to the pharynx. An external air bypass and a pseudolarynx mechanism is inserted between the tracheostoma and the fistula. The vibrating mechanism uses a rubber reed

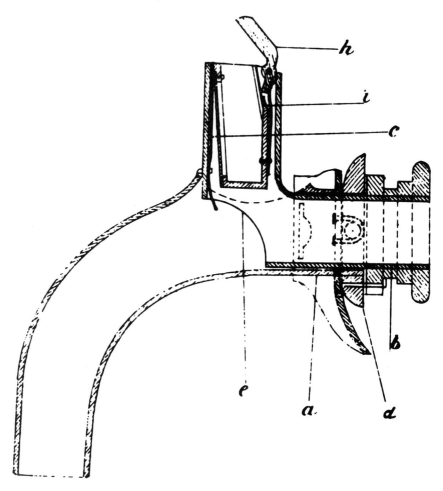

Figure 6-11. Artificial larynx developed by Josef Leiter, 1873. (Reprinted with permission. *The Artificial Larynx.* Yvan Lebrun. Swets and Zeitlinger, B.V. Amsterdam 1973.)

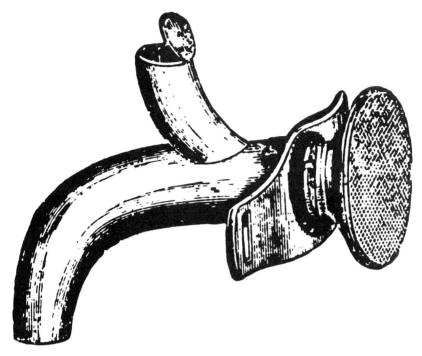

Figure 6-12. Artificial larynx developed by Carl Gussenbauer, 1874. (Reprinted with permission. *The Artificial Larynx.* Yvan Lebrun. Swets and Zeitlinger, B.V. Amsterdam 1973.)

similar to the Tokyo artificial larynx (*see* Fig. 6-16).

The Northwestern Voice Prosthesis was developed by Sisson and his colleagues (1975). This device contains no vibrator, but achieves voicing by the placement of a pharyngostoma, which can be surgically made at the time of the laryngectomy. The placement of this stoma is most critical in order to achieve voicing. An appliance is inserted between the tracheostoma and

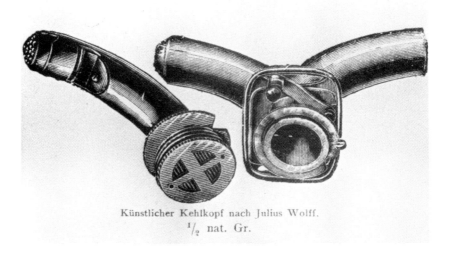

Künstlicher Kehlkopf nach Julius Wolff.

$^1/_2$ nat. Gr.

Figure 6-13. Artificial larynx developed by Julius Wolf, 1893. (Reprinted with permission. *The Artificial Larynx*. Yvan Lebrun. Swets and Zeitlinger, B.V. Amsterdam 1973.)

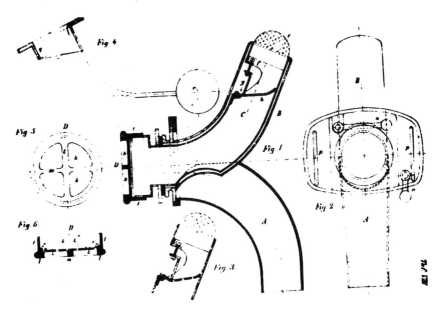

Figure 6-14. Schematic of artificial larynx developed by Julius Wolf. (Reprinted with permission. *The Artificial Larynx*. Yvan Lebrun. Swets and Zeitlinger, B.V. Amsterdam 1973.)

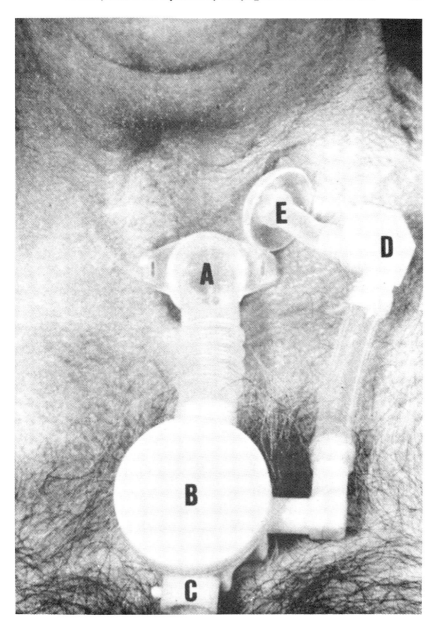

Figure 6-15. LaBarge VoiceBak prosthesis. *A.* Tracheal interconnector. *B.* Bypass valve. *C.* Breathing port. *D.* Fistula valve. *E.* Flanged fistula tube. (Reprinted with permission. *The Artificial Larynx Handbook.* Salmon and Goldstein, eds. Grune and Stratton, N.Y. 1978.)

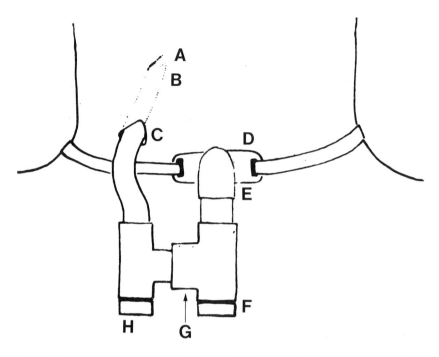

Figure 6-16. Reed-fistula appliance. *A.* Inner valve. *B.* Fistula tube. *C.* Fistula. *D.* Tracheostomy tube. *E.* Tracheal connector. *F.* Inspiratory valve. *G.* Reed housing. *H.* Saliva trap. (Reprinted with permission. *The Artificial Larynx Handbook.* Salmon and Goldstein, eds. Grune and Stratton, N.Y. 1978.)

the pharyngostoma. It contains a valve that can be set at various pulmonary pressure levels that allows for breathing, coughing, and speech production (*see* Fig 6-17).

Most recently, Singer and Blom (1980) have reported on their tracheoesophageal puncture—a surgical-prosthetic technique for postlaryngectomy speech restoration. This procedure consists of surgically producing a puncture at the twelve o'clock position in the tracheostoma leading to the esophagus. A "duckbill" prosthesis (*see* Fig. 6-18) is inserted, and through digital closure of the stoma, air is diverted into the esophagus (*see* Fig. 6-19).

These devices all have the advantage of using pulmonary air for voicing, thereby leading to a more natural method of speech production.

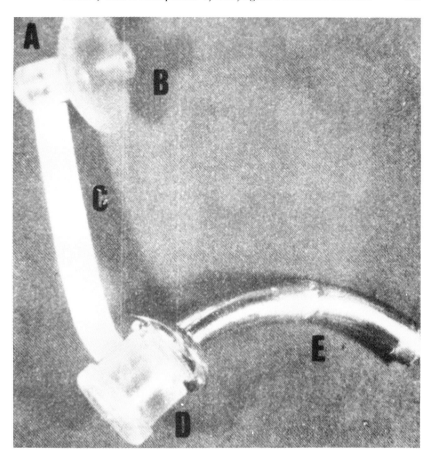

Figure 6-17. Northwestern voice prosthesis. *A*. One-way valve. *B*. Fistula fitting. *C*. Conduit. *D*. Respiratory valve. *E*. Tracheal connector. (Reprinted with permission. *The Artificial Larynx Handbook.* Salmon and Goldstein, eds. Grune and Stratton, N.Y. 1978.)

Compared to esophageal speakers, individuals using these types of devices can usually talk for longer periods of time, produce more words per air intake, and generally talk faster and achieve a more natural voice quality. For those devices that have a pulmonary valve for voice, the idea of spontaneity of speech is greatly enhanced. The patient does not have to worry about the placement of a finger for closure in order to produce short responses.

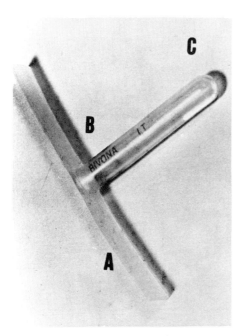

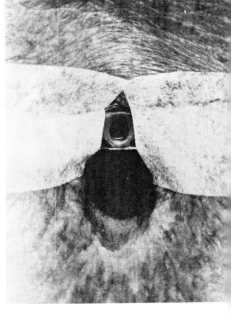

Figure 6-18. Blom-Singer voice prosthesis. *A.* Retention flange. *B.* Air entry. *C.* One-way valved end.

Figure 6-19. Blom-Singer voice prosthesis in place.

Users of the early devices had to exercise care because of the danger of complication of leakage and possible aspiration. The newer surgical techniques have greatly eliminated the danger of aspiration but continue to have leakage problems from the fistulas, which become embarrassing and annoying to the patient. Patients also complain of having to take care of two stomas now rather than one. Finally, the external pneumatic devices, such as the Tokyo, although the quality has been rated as superior to other devices, requires the patient to talk while having a tube inserted in the oral cavity. This usually interferes with the overall articulation quality for most patients, as well as being aesthetically embarrassing.

Electrolarynges

The first electrolarynx was developed by Gluck around 1909, and it consisted of an Edison-type phonograph cylinder containing vowel sounds. These sounds were dampened and fed through a receiver that was inserted in the patient's nose. It is very possible that this device was the reason that the electrolarynx really did not appear on the market until the 1950s.

Tait, in 1959, reported the development of a denture-mounted electrolarynx. The initial prototype of the "oral vibrator" consisted of an electromagnetic diaphragm concealed in the center of an upper denture. A wire was led out of the mouth to a small box containing a battery-powered, transistorized audio-oscillator. A second prototype eliminated the manually activated switch, battery pack, and wire leading out of the mouth. The on-off switch was accomplished by pressure exerted on specific areas of the prosthesis. The batteries were charged when the dental plate was not being worn (*see* Fig. 6-20). The vocal quality was

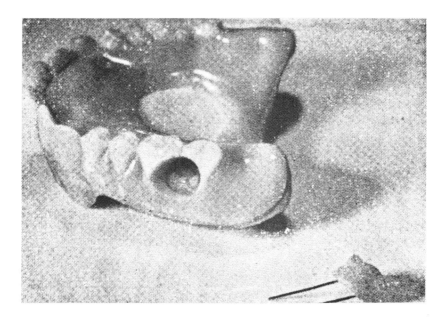

Figure 6-20. Tait's "Oral Vibrator". (Reprinted with permission. *British Dental Journal, 109*:507, 1960.)

extremely mechanical, and the individual was unable to produce an /h/ or a / ŋ / sound.

It is obvious that the quality of the sound produced by these devices depends on the nature of the generated pulse. F. Firestone had the idea of using an air-filled tube to deliver the generated pulses into the speaker's mouth, and this device was manufactured by Cooper-Rand Company (*see* Fig. 6-21). With this device, the oscillator is powered by a battery, and the pulses are directed into the oral cavity through a small plastic tube. Although there are controls to alter the frequency and the intensity, the overall tonal quality remains mechanical. There is also the problem of articulation with the tube in the oral cavity.

In an attempt to conceal the electromagnetic vibrator, Ticchioni

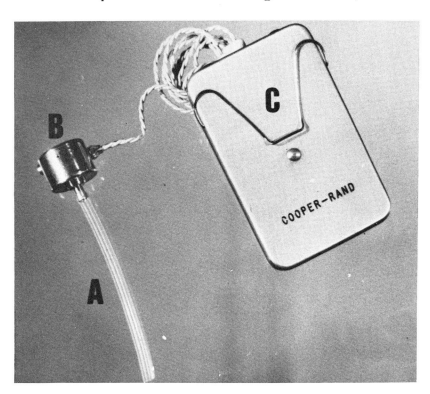

Figure 6-21. Cooper Rand artificial larynx. A. Mouth-tube. B. Tone generator. C. Pulse generator and battery case. (Reprinted with permission. *The Artificial Larynx Handbook.* Salmon and Goldstein, eds. Grune and Stratton, N.Y. 1978.)

placed it within the bowl of a pipe (*see* Fig. 6-22). The pulses traveled through the stem of the pipe directly into the oral cavity.

In the late 1950s with the introduction of the transistor, the transcervical electronic larynx was developed. There are currently four of these devices on the market. They are:

1. The Western Electric No. 5A and 5B, which features a pitch manipulator (*see* Fig. 6-23);
2. The Aurex Neovox, with comes with rechargeable batteries (*see* Fig. 6-24);
3. The Servox Electric larynx, also with rechargeable batteries and intensity/frequency switches (*see* Fig. 6-25); and
4. The Barts vibrator electronic larynx (*see* Fig. 6-26).

These devices vary mainly in the manner used to produce sound. As shown in Figure 6-27, the Western Electric uses an electromagnetic sound source, the Aurex uses a solenoid, the Servox uses a voice coil, and the Barts uses a rectilinear oscillation system.

Each of these devices, although widely used, have many limitations. First, they all produce mechanical vocal quality. This is even true for the devices with the ability to manipulate and change the pitch. They are all required to be held in the hand in order to be coupled with neck tissue. This creates two problems:

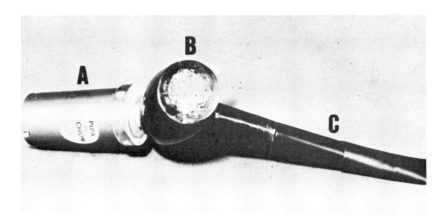

Figure 6-22. Ticchioni pipe artificial larynx. A. Battery. B. Tone generator. C. Mouth-tube. (Reprinted with permission. *The Artificial Larynx Handbook.* Salmon and Goldstein, eds. Grune and Stratton, N.Y. 1978.)

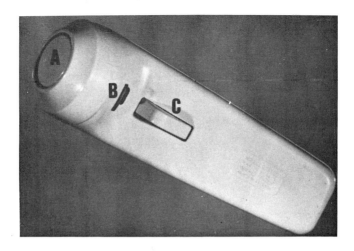

Figure 6-23. Western Electric 5A artificial larynx. A. Sound source. B. Power switch. C. Pitch control. (Reprinted with permission. *The Artificial Larynx Handbook*. Salmon and Goldstein, eds. Grune and Stratton, N.Y. 1978.)

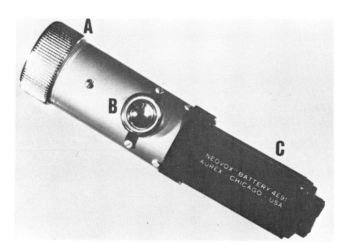

Figure 6-24. Aurex Neovox artificial larynx. A. Vibratory mechanism. B. On-off switch. C. Rechargeable battery. (Reprinted with permission. *The Artificial Larynx Handbook*. Salmon and Goldstein, eds. Grune and Stratton, N.Y. 1978.)

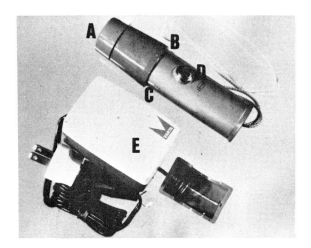

Figure 6-25. Servox artificial larynx. A. Vibratory
mechanism. B. Pitch control. C. Volume control. D.
On-off switch. E. Battery charger. (Reprinted with
permission. *The Artificial Larynx Handbook.* Salmon
and Goldstein, eds. Grune and Stratton, N.Y. 1978.)

(1) having to constantly move the hand to the neck and (2)
holding it there becomes tiring and tedious. Individuals tend to
eliminate casual remarks because of this effort. In order to achieve
maximum quality, complete coupling must take place between
the neck tissue and the device. This is not always achieved with
every attempt at speaking. It should also be noted that all of these
devices create external-competing noise, sometimes calling more
attention to the sound than the speech.

Two of the devices (the Western Electric and the Aurex) have
the capability of being modified for use as an intraoral-prosthetic
device. These include: the Creech modification (*see* Fig. 6-28);
the Williams and Ostray modification (*see* Fig. 6-29), with the
use of a hearing aid receiver; the Zwitman and Disinger modification (*see* Fig. 6-30), also using a hearing aid receiver; and the
commercially available Aurex-Neovox M-550 cap (Fig. 6-31).

Recently there has been a resurgence of interest in the
development and improvement of electronic artificial larynges;
they have taken many directions, including implantation. Some

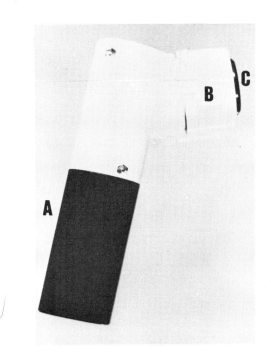

Figure 6-26. Barts vibrator artificial larynx. A. Battery. B. Locking ring. C. Vibratory mechanism. (Reprinted with permission. *The Artificial Larynx Handbook.* Salmon and Goldstein, eds. Grune and Stratton, N.Y. 1978.)

SOUND SOURCE

WESTERN ELECTRIC 5A	---	ELECTROMAGNETIC
AUREX NEOVOX	---	SOLENOID
SERVOX	---	VOICE COIL
BARTS	---	RECTILINEAR OSCILLATION

Figure 6-27. Sound source of the transcervical artificial larynx.

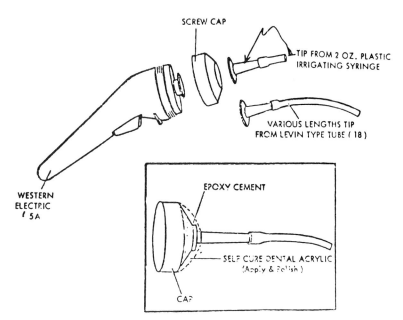

Figure 6-28. Creech modification of the Western Electric 5A. (Reprinted with permission. *The Artificial Larynx Handbook*. Salmon and Goldstein, eds. Grune and Stratton, N.Y. 1978.)

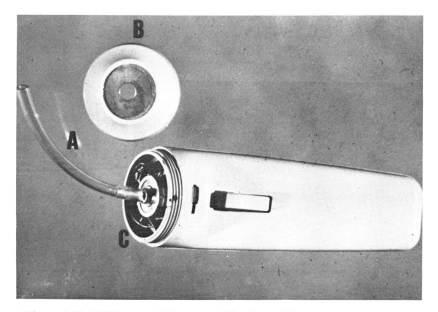

Figure 6-29. Williams and Ostray modification of the Western Electric 5A. A. Mouth-tube. B. Cap with cover plate. C. Body-type hearing aid receiver. (Reprinted with permission. *The Artificial Larynx Handbook*. Salmon and Goldstein, eds. Grune and Stratton, N.Y. 1978.)

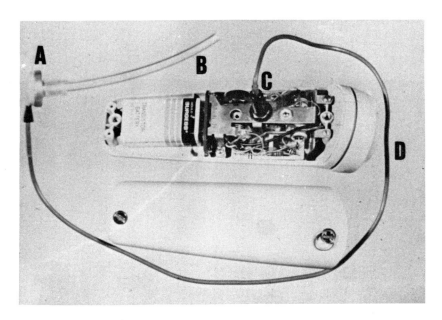

Figure 6-30. Zwitman and Disinger modification of the Western Electric 5A. A. Body-type hearing aid receiver. B. Mouth-tube. C. Shorting jack and plug. D. Cord. (Reprinted with permission. *The Artificial Larynx Handbook.* Salmon and Goldstein, eds. Grune and Stratton, N.Y. 1978.)

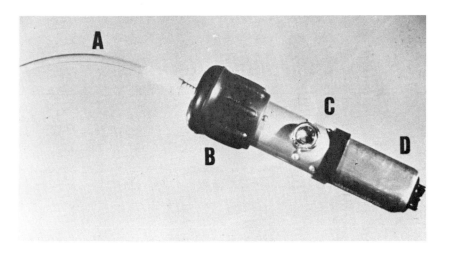

Figure 6-31. Aurex Neovox M-550. A. Mouth-tube. B. M-550 cap. C. Vibrator mechanism. D. Rechargeable battery. (Reprinted with permission. *The Artificial Larynx Handbook.* Salmon and Goldstein, eds. Grune and Stratton, N.Y. 1978.)

of these new devices that are currently being developed are reported elsewhere in this volume and, therefore, are not included in this discussion.

Goldstein, Rothman, and Oliver (1978) have been investigating the development of a new artificial larynx since 1978. The goals of this program have been to develop a neck-mounted vibration device that (1) is cosmetically pleasing; (2) has effective contact over a wide range of postsurgical anatomical structures; (3) can be fitted to the neck for extended periods of time; (4) has a choice of activation by either resistive respiratory pressure, muscle action potential or hand switch; (5) will be highly intelligible over a wide range of acoustic environments; and (6) will be driven by a waveform similar to the natural laryngeal tone. The prototype device (*see* Fig. 6-32) is one of balanced rotational oscillation. The rotating crank on the motor drives a small rotor (set in bearings) in oscillatory motion through 10-15 degrees. A shaft is inserted in the rotor at one end and has an impactor mass at the other end. The impactor mass strikes a soft-palate disc that is coupled to the neck and held in place by a collar, which helps to attenuate masking transmission and reduce power requirements. The system is battery powered and is still undergoing modifications (*see* Fig. 6-33). Presently the device compares favorably to the existing devices.

SUMMARY

Current approaches to artificial larynx improvement are continuing in a twofold direction, and there is still considerable work being accomplished in the area of pneumatic devices. These have taken on the direction of incorporating surgical and prosthetic techniques. In response to the newest technique by Singer and Blom (1980), Dr. Cantrell reports that the procedure is a major step forward, but we should have no illusions that this is the end of the road in pseudoglottic voice restoration.

There is also major research and development in the area of electroacoustical devices. In reviewing various artificial larynges, in 1975 Goode concluded that the ideal artificial larynx had not yet been developed. This statement may still be true, but with the

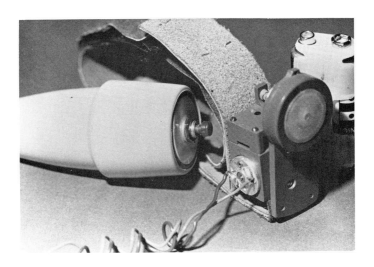

Figure 6-32. Prototype of a neck-mounted artificial larynx. Developed by Goldstein, Rothman, and Oliver at the VA Medical Center and University of Florida, Gainesville, Florida.

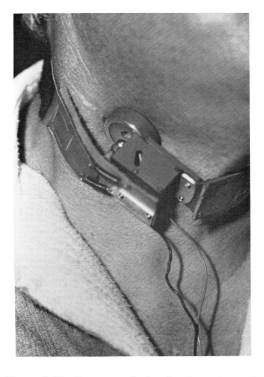

Figure 6-33. Prototype device fitted on the neck.

electroacoustical and bioengineering research currently being accomplished we are getting closer to the ideal artificial larynx.

REFERENCES

Goldstein, L.P.: Historical review of the artificial larynx. *V.A. Southeastern REMC Proceedings.* Birmingham, Alabama, 1976.

Goldstein, L.P., Rothman, H.B., and Oliver, C.: Development and evaluation of a new artificial larynx. *Bull Prosthetics Research, 10-29:*186, 1978.

Goode, R.L.: Artificial laryngeal devices in post-laryngectomy rehabilitation. *Laryngoscope, 85:*677-689, 1975.

Lebrun, Y.: *The Artificial Larynx.* Amsterdam: Swets and Zeitlinger B.V., 1973.

Nelson, I.W., Parkin, J.L., and Potter, J.F.: The modified Tokyo larynx. *Arch Otolaryngol, 101:*107-108, 1975.

Salmon, S.J., and Goldstein, L.P. *The Artificial Larynx Handbook.* New York: Grune, 1978.

Shedd, D., Bakajan, V., Sako, K., Mann, M., Weinberg B., and Schaaf, N.: Reed-fistula method of speech rehabilitation after laryngectomy. *Am J Surg, 124:* 510-514, 1972.

Singer, M.I., and Blom, E.D.: *An Endoscopic Technique for Restoration of Voice after Laryngectomy.* Presented at the Annual Meeting of the American Laryngologic Assoc., Inc., Palm Beach, Fl., April 15, 1980.

Sisson, G.A., McConnel, F.M.S., Logeman, J.A., and Yeh, S., Jr.: Voice rehabilitation after laryngectomy. *Arch Otolaryngol, 101:*178-181, 1975.

Weinberg, B., and Riekena, A.: Speech produced with the Tokyo artificial larynx. *J Speech Hear Disord, 38:*383-389, 1973.

Weinberg, B., Shedd, D.P., and Horii, Y.: Reed-fistula speech following pharyngolaryngectomy. *J Speech Hear Disord, 43:*401-413, 1978.

LARYNGECTOMEE SPEECH SUPPORT SYSTEM WITH PROSODIC CONTROL

ANDREW SEKEY AND ROBERT HANSON

ABSTRACT

Design principles of a hands-free, variable-pitch, controlled-volume, unobtrusive speech support system for laryngectomees are described. The scheme is to make efficient use of residual articulatory faculties of laryngectomees and to exploit digital signal processing techniques and devices. The following novel features characterize the system now being developed:

1. The vocal tract is excited by a miniature, low-power driver affixed inside the oral cavity; ensuing sound is sensed by an intraoral miniature acoustic sensor.
2. Control and information signals to and from the mouth are transmitted by electromagnetic coupling.
3. Actual speech sounds are radiated, after amplification and spectral correction, from a chest-level concealed loudspeaker.
4. Intonation and dynamics are regulated by the speaker through the rate of exhalation, which is sensed by a miniature device positioned at the stoma opening.

INTRODUCTION

THE LONG-TERM GOAL of this ongoing project is to develop a hands-free, variable-pitch, controlled-volume, unobtrusive speech support system for laryngectomees.

Such a system, whose installation would at most require minor

Most of the work reported here has been performed under Grant No. PDT-113 of the American Cancer Society, Inc. Valuable contributions to various phases of the project were made by Karen Doyle, Jon Forrest, Steven Hiller, and Charles Seagrave. We are grateful to Knowles Electronics, Inc., for the gift of sample transducers.

surgery, is envisioned to incorporate an intraoral sound source and sensor, radio communication between the oral cavity and body-worn equipment, sophisticated digital processing of components of the enhanced speech signal, and external amplification of sound. Consequently, in this research we have been exploring the effects on speech of nonconventional excitation of the vocal tract, as well as the precision with which humans can control the rate of their breath flow. The objective of the latter is to derive time-varying analog control signals for pitch and intensity from tracheal airflow rate, a novel idea whose feasibility has been demonstrated in preliminary studies.

Some of the fundamental research associated with these objectives may also be of value in other health-related fields, such as in mobility and communication aids for the severely disabled and in phonation disorders not requiring laryngectomy.

RATIONALE FOR THE SYSTEM UNDER DEVELOPMENT

The starting premise of this project was that by exploiting recent advances in the understanding of speech acoustics and in speech-signal processing it might be possible to combine the medical simplicity of intraoral vibrators (e.g. Knorr and Zwitman 1977; Zwitman et al. 1977) with the acoustic advantage (as argued by its proponents) of implanted artificial larynges (*see* Chapter 12). As regards the latter, we note that it is becoming increasingly cheaper to provide sophisticated electronic prostheses, whilst the cost of surgery, hospitalization, and postoperative treatment rises constantly. Moreover, patients cannot always sustain additional surgery immediately after undergoing laryngectomy. These factors provide strong motivation for finding a technological alternative to implantation into the pharyngeal wall. *Transcervical vibrators* (*see* Chapter 6) have several intrinsic limitations, such as back radiation, high visibility, and their unsuitability for patients with scarred or hardened neck tissue (Zwitman and Disinger 1975), some of which may never be overcome. *Oral vibrators* thus provide the logical alternative.

A basic problem with an oral vibrator is that no matter where it is installed, its location differs from that of the larynx it replaces. Consequently, the resonant pattern set up by its vibration in the vocal tract would, generally, also differ from the natural pattern. When this difference becomes noticeable, it contributes to the unnatural sound of the speech and decreases intelligibility. A further limitation of oral vibrators is the low level of their undistorted power output, due to the necessarily small size. This is particularly noticed outdoors or in a noisy environment.

Both problems might be resolved by placing inside the mouth a miniature sound sensor, whose output would be processed to reduce distortions and amplified to provide sufficient acoustic power. Furthermore, the intraoral sensor developed for a fully artificial system might also be of value for *esophageal speakers*. In fact, there is no reason why even the vibrator-plus-sensor system could not beneficially co-exist with a limited degree of esophageal speech, the latter providing the air necessary for fricatives and plosives, and the former augmenting the vowel production with variable pitch as an added feature.

In order to improve the intelligibility and naturalness of the semi-synthetic speech generated by the use of such a prosthesis it is necessary to provide for the modulation of pitch and intensity. None of the commercial devices and only a few experimental ones presently attempt to do this, usually by manual control (*see* Chapter 8) possibly combined with preprogramming (*see* Chapter 9). Our approach is to utilize the pulmonary airflow at the stoma by deriving from it the appropriate control signals, the feasibility of which will be discussed next. This would restore to the respiratory system, albeit in a modified form, the role it plays in speech production, while freeing the user's hands for other purposes.

The focal areas of our research towards realizing the ultimate goal of a working system thus are:

1. Study of the types of distortion encountered in the speech signal and possible methods for their correction, when the phonating source is (instead of at the glottis) somewhere in front of the oral cavity, and the resultant sound is sensed intraorally

2. Selection of an intraoral driver and sound sensor to meet the physical and environmental requirements of the given

task, and experimentation with alternative methods of attaching them within the oral cavity

3. Development of a miniature sensor for airflow that can be mounted within a stoma button, and exploration of users' ability to regulate tracheal airflow accurately enough to serve as control signal for pitch and intensity

4. Development of methods of energy transfer, modulation, and coding by which the intraoral devices can be effectively linked to body-worn equipment.

OVERALL DESCRIPTION OF THE SYSTEM

Our current conception of the prototype system, whose design would be based on findings of ongoing research, can be described as the interconnection of the following subsystems:

a. Pulmonary airflow sensor (over the stoma)
b. Excitation signal generator and transmitter
c. External (neck) antenna loop
d. Internal (oral) antenna loop
e. Receiver and electroacoustic driver (intraorally mounted)
f. Acoustic sensor and signal transmitter (intraorally mounted)
g. Signal processor and power amplifier
h. Loudspeaker (worn over the chest)
i. Battery pack

The physical layout of these components is illustrated in Figure 7-1 and their interconnections in Figure 7-2.

Operation of the System

Activated by the pulmonary airflow sensor (a), the excitation generator (b) produces a substitute larynx tone that is modulated onto a high-frequency carrier and then radiated by the external antenna (c). Part of the radiated energy is picked up by the internal antenna (d) and is converted to an acoustic signal by the intraorally mounted electroacoustic driver (e). The sound so created is selectively amplified by the vocal cavity and may be augmented by fricative and plosive sounds produced by buccal or esophageal air.

The aggregate speech sounds are sensed by the intraoral

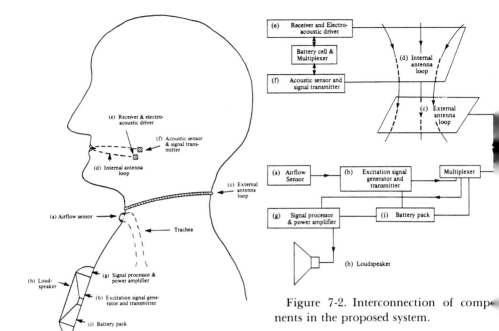

Figure 7-2. Interconnection of components in the proposed system.

Figure 7-1. Physical layout of the proposed system.

accoustic sensor (f), which then modulates them onto a different carrier from that used before and re-radiates them through the same internal antenna (d). The signal picked up by the external antenna (c) is electronically processed and amplified by the signal processor (g) and is then radiated at an adjustable average power level through the loudspeaker (h). Power for external components is provided by the battery pack (i).

At first sight this may seem a forbiddingly complex system; however, most components are either available off-the-shelf or can be modified from available items. The main problem areas are signal processing and prosthetics. (The latter refers to methods of mounting the transducers—e.g. artificial palate, dentures, implantation—protecting them from environmental hazards, biocompatibility, etc.)

We also foresee an alternative mode of operation (Sekey 1980) that would be invoked if no effective methods were found to correct, in real time, spectral distortions engendered by the intraoral system. In this mode the role of the intraoral driver is limited to the generation of a wide-band "sounding" signal for the tract. The output of the sensor is then processed to yield an estimate of tract parameters, which in turn are used to control a separate speech synthesizer. This would thus essentially be an unconventional input vocoder.

It may be feared that prospective users would become self-conscious about their amplified voice emerging from a flat loudspeaker strapped to their chest. However, disparity between the assumed visual and actual sources of sound is already present for laryngectomees using a shirt-pocket amplifier, as well as in every television set.

In what follows we shall discuss in some detail three aspects of our scheme: airflow control, intraoral sound fields, and transducers.

AIRFLOW CONTROL OF PITCH

As is well known (e.g. Titze 1974), in "normal" speech the fundamental frequency (f_0) is determined by a delicate interplay of laryngeal muscle activity and subglottal air pressure, the latter originating in pulmonary activity. While in normal speech the lungs function essentially only as a power supply or "tank circuit," they can assume a more independent role in singing and in the playing of wind instruments. These facts encouraged us to experiment with the use of airflow as a control signal.

In our first set of experiments the subject received visual feedback from an oscilloscope screen, which displayed both a "target" curve and the time variations of his own breath flow. A detailed description has appeared elsewhere (Sekey 1978*a*) and will not be repeated here.

In a second set of tests the feedback was auditory, and the subject aimed at mimicking the intonation pattern of a short utterance recorded on an endless tape loop. The experimental arrangement is shown in Figure 7-3. The subject, a twenty-three-year-old female graduate student, was a native English speaker. She first recorded several test sentences, which were then passed

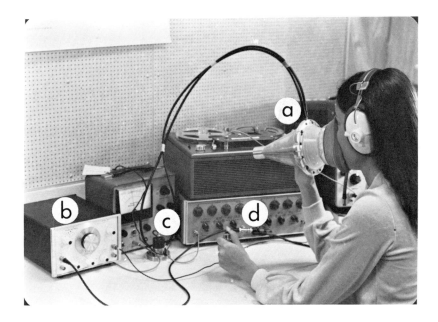

Figure 7-3. Experimental arrangement of airflow experiments: (a) pneumotachograph; (b) voltage-controlled oscillator (c) pressure transducer and differential amplifier; and (d) low-pass filter.

through a Frøker-Jensen Trans-Pitchmeter®. The resulting pitch contours were recorded on endless tape loops, and she listened to these in one ear while in the other ear she heard a triangular carrier wave whose pitch was proportional to her rate of exhalation. Pitch imitation contours resulting from typical experiments are shown in Figure 7-4. They compare favorably (except for a lack of time normalization) with a similar set derived from actual speech signals (Jassem 1975).

In the next phase of our experiments we employed a similar setup but for controlling the f_o input to a Computalker® model CT-1 Speech Synthesizer. Test sentences representing a variety of intonation patterns were synthesized on the Computalker, and the subject was familiarized with their rhythm by listening to them. Next, the Computalker's f_o control signal was replaced by one derived from the subject's airflow. After a short practice, fairly natural sounding intonation patterns were generated. (A

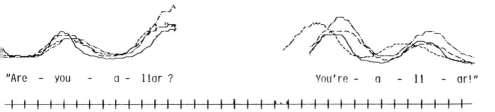

"Are - you - ɑ - llar ?   You're - ɑ - ll - ɑr!"

Figure 7-4. Airflow-controlled imitations of pitch contours: solid line—reference (output pitch meter); dot/dash line—first imitation (without practice); short dashes line—second imitation (after 20 minutes practice); and long dashes line—third imitation (after 30 minutes practice)

Horizontal scale: 0.1 seconds/division
Vertical scale: linear in frequency

tape comparing these with the Computalker's own program-mable intonation patterns was played at the conference; a copy may be requested from Dr. Sekey.)

The pneumotachograph has proved itself a valuable research tool, but is impractical for converting stomal airflow into a control signal, as prescribed by our scheme. We thus developed a practical alternative: a thermistor-based airflow sensing system. This is sufficiently small to be built into a stoma button, yet can be made linear enough to produce the required control signal. A detailed description appears elsewhere (Sekey and Seagrave 1981).

Occasional interference with the pitch control is expected from the user coughing or clearing his stoma. Coughing produces a "burst-like"exhalation, and a threshold could be set in the signal amplifier to recognize and ignore it. Clearing the stoma could present a problem for the airflow sensor. In the final implemen-tation it may be necessary to make the sensor readily removable for this purpose.

Intensity Control

While the above discussion is limited to the control of *pitch* through airflow, our scheme actually calls for the control of *intensity* as well. These two parameters are generally known to be related (e.g. Lieberman 1967), though we are not aware of any practical exploitation of their relationship. To highlight this dependence, we collected data on five sentences of different type, each spoken by five different speakers.

The sentences were recorded on a Nagra model IVD tape recorder at 15 ips. They were subsequently low-pass filtered by a Krohn Hite model 3322 low-pass filter ("maximally flat" setting) and digitized at 12,000 samples/per second.

Pitch and intensity contours were obtained by using the Interactive Laboratory System (ILS)® speech signal-processing software package developed by Signal Technology, Inc. The specific subroutine employed has been described by Juang and Markel (1979). It is a robust, modified homomorphic pitch detector in which voiced/unvoiced decisions are made on the basis of five parameters, followed by the extraction (when applicable) of a pitch parameter. (In the absence of voicing, the original package produces a preset level, but we modified it to leave the f_0 plot blank.)

At 12,000 samples/s the 256 sample analysis frames correspond to 21.3 ms, i.e. 2-3 pitch periods. Consecutive frames overlapped by 120 samples (or 10 ms). Each analysis stage yields one estimated value of f_0 so that the density of points in the pitch contours to be presented is 100 points/s.

Since the human ear responds approximately to the *logarithm* of frequency, we shall show plots of the base two logarithms of the ratio of extracted f_0 values to the starting value of f_0, sometimes called "octave numbers." Any other choice of reference frequency and base of logarithm would, of course, only effect a linear transformation on the contours.

The intensity curves were derived from instantaneous rms values yielded by an ILS routine. Two further operations were performed: first, the logarithm of the raw values was taken for the same psychoacoustic reason as for pitch; and second, the values so obtained were averaged by a five-point "boxcar" integrator, i.e. each plotted value is actually the mean of two neighbors on each side, plus itself. This step was found necessary because the original fluctuations in the raw values, which were rather more rapid than those of the f_0 curve, are disturbing and irrelevant in the study of pitch-intensity relations. The choice of the averaging period was arrived at by trial and error.

A typical example is shown in Figure 7-5. The sentence, "We were away a year ago," was spoken by an American male subject. It confirms the expected similarities as well as some differences (especially at the word-boundary "we were" and at the end of the sentence), yet is very suggestive of the possibility of deriving both pitch and intensity contours from the same control signal.

VOCAL-TRACT MODELLING

Modelling the vocal tract by mechanical, electrical, and mathematical models is already a well-established art (Fant 1960; Flanagan 1972). More recent digital methods (Markel and Gray 1976) permit the computation of area ratios in an acoustic-tube

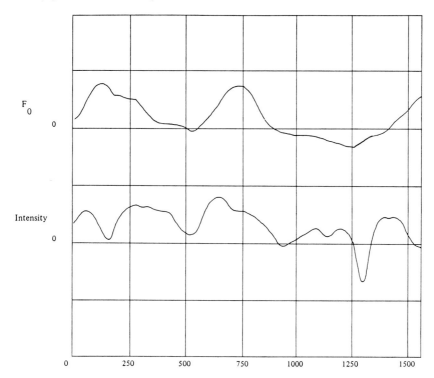

Figure 7-5. Fundamental frequency (f_0) and intensity contours of the sentence "We were away a year ago" spoken by an American male.
Horizontal scale: milliseconds
Vertical divisions: 1 octave for f_0; 10 db for intensity

equivalent of the vocal tract through parameters extracted from the speech waveform. All these models assume, however, that the tract is excited at the larynx, *and* that sound propagates along the tube in one-dimensional plane waves.* This assumption is reasonably good for the wavelengths of interest in speech.

With the tract excited somewhere along its length by a small, point-like source, which may be located away from the axis of lateral symmetry, the resulting wave pattern will generally be complex, and plane wave propagation cannot be assumed. When the sensor, too, is placed intraorally, and not necessarily at a location in any way symmetrical to the source, the mathematics become intractable. An analytic approach thus seems unpromising; instead, we have chosen to work on three levels of modeling, increasing in realism:

Level 1: computer simulation of the vocal tract

Level 2: mechanical model of the vocal tract

Level 3: actual vocal tract

Level 1 requires the most abstraction, but is not far removed from the mathematical description and offers the advantage of combined "experimentation" and calculation (e.g. of measures of error or efficiency.)

Level 2 possesses the realism of actual transducers and sensors and an (albeit crude) approximation to a physical vocal tract.

Level 3 is most realistic but least amenable to predictions and optimization.

In modelling the vocal tract of a laryngectomee, one must also take into account the change in glottal-boundary conditions resulting from the removal of the larynx, as well as articulatory compensation (Weinberg 1980; *see also* Chapter 1). Further, if an intraoral prosthesis is anticipated, as in our scheme, it *may* also noticeably affect the resonant properties of the vocal cavity.

While we did run tests on Level 1, using the VOCALT acoustic-tube computer simulation program, analysis of the results is still in progress and will not be reported here. Instead,

---

*Excitation by a source forward in the tract is discussed by Flanagan (1972), in connection with fricative generation. Plane-wave propagation is still presumed, and it is found that (unlike for glottal excitation) the forward transmission has zeros at several frequencies, though some of these are cancelled out by close-lying poles.

we shall briefly describe experiments conducted at the other two levels.

Mechanical Model of the Vocal Tract

Experiments were performed on a mechanical model of the vocal tract, which was constructed in-house to our specifications. Figures 7-6 and 7-7 show the tract and its sound-absorbent

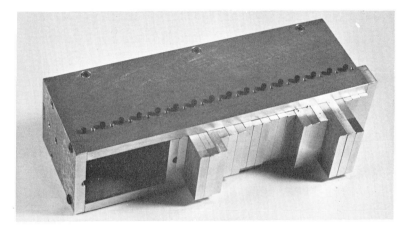

Figure 7-6. Frontal view of the vocal-tract model adjusted for the vowel /u/.

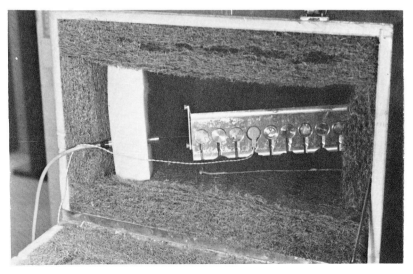

Figure 7-7. Rear view of the vocal-tract model prepared for measurement in soundproof housing.

housing during testing. It consists of a rectangular tube, whose interior cross section can be varied stepwise along its axis by sliding the slabs that form one side of the tube. One dimension of the internal cross section is thus constant (5 cm), while the other may be continuously varied from 0 to 5 cm. The slabs are 8 mm thick, so that the 25.6 cm long tract can house up to 32 of them. Provision is made for the insertion of a standard hearing-aid earphone at the terminating slab or at one of the 10 side-openings spaced uniformly at 25.4 mm intervals along the tube (cf. Fig. 7-7). In the experiments, tracts consisting either of 21 slabs (16.8 cm) or 15 slabs (12 cm) were used.

In addition to moving the source, we could also sense the sound field at various cross sections of the tract by inserting a B & K microphone probe.

Of the numerous experiments performed (cf. e.g. Sekey 1978*b*), we only show here one set of typical results in which transfer functions of the vocal tract with seven different source locations are superimposed in a pseudo-three-dimensional picture (*see* Figure 7-8). The original formant pattern is seen to undergo

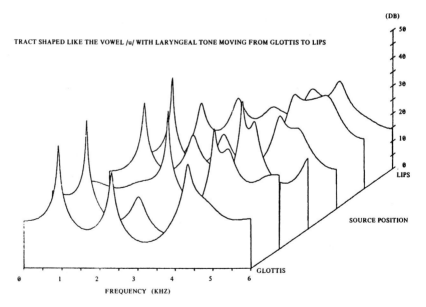

Figure 7-8. Variations in simulated formant pattern with driver moving from "glottis" to "lips" in mechanical-tract model.

considerable variations as the source progresses along the tract. Complementary measurements were made with the sensor moving while the source remains stationary. The goal of such experiments is to determine the best source/sensor position within the mouth for correctability of distortions.

Intraoral Experiments with Miniature Transducers

At the highest level of realism one must work with an actual vocal tract, and so we placed miniature transducers (a driver and a microphone) into subjects' (two of the investigators) mouths and measured resultant changes in formant patterns. The microphone was a Knowles type EA 1842 (dimensions 4.0 x 5.6 x 2.3 mm), and the driver was Knowles type ED 1912 "Receiver" (dimensions 4.3 x 6.3 x 3.0 mm).

When used intraorally, both transducers were imbedded in dental wax and attached to an individual artificial palate prepared by a dental consultant. The layout is shown in Figure 7-9. Prior to insertion in the palate the output of the driver corresponding to an imitation glottal pulse (8 ms period, 1:4 duty cycle) was measured under four different conditions: in "free field" (i.e. in the soundproof box seen in Figure 7-7), with both a B & K ½" condenser microphone and the Knowles miniature microphone, and by a B & K 2 cm³ coupler, again with both

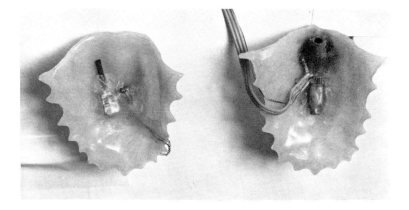

Figure 7-9. Intraoral transducers mounted in artificial palates by different methods.

microphones. Data files thus created were subsequently used for inverse filtering so as to eliminate the effects of transducer distortion.

In initial exploratory tests we obtained spectra for the vowels /ɑ/, /i/, and /u/ while permuting all the experimental variables as follows:

1. Natural phonation, condenser microphone 10 cm from mouth
2. Natural phonation, miniature microphone 10 cm from mouth
3. Natural phonation, miniature microphone in palate
4. Intraoral driver, condenser microphone 2 cm from mouth
5. Intraoral driver, miniature microphone 2 cm from mouth
6. Intraoral driver, miniature microphone in palate

Two of the eighteen resulting spectra are shown in Figure 7-10.

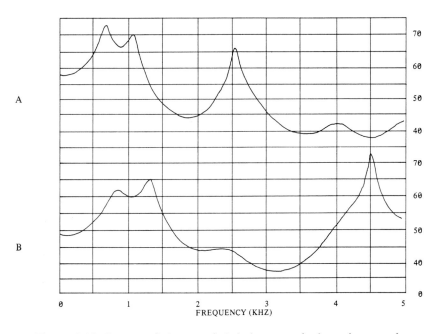

Figure 7-10. Spectra of the vowel /ɑ/; A—natural phonation; condenser microphone 10 cm from mouth; and B—excitation by intraoral driver, sensing by intraoral miniature microphone.

Curve A—condition (1)—is a fairly good representation of a natural /ɑ/; in curve B—condition (6)—we see the almost total disappearance of the third formant accompanied by shifts in amplitude and intensity of the first two formants. The former effect seems to be due to the intraoral microphone being in a nodal position for the third formant. Note also the overwhelming resonance at 4.5 kHz. This is also present, to a lesser extent, for the other two vowels in condition (b).

Another unconventional element in our system is the flat, chest-mounted loudspeaker. It is only fairly recently that commercial varieties have become available: Figure 7-11 shows a sample we acquired from the PolyPlanar company; this is not the smallest available type, but gives a fair idea of what we would use.

SUMMARY

We see the main significance of our system under development in the breadth of its attack on the problem of speech aids. Instead of merely improving on the concept of an "artificial larynx," we

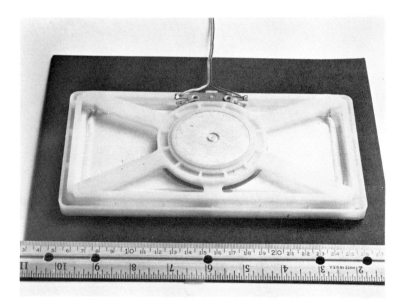

Figure 7-11. Typical ultra-slim loudspeaker (Poly-Planar P-5B) suitable for concealed wear over the chest.

intend to lay the foundations of a systematic approach to a broad class of phonatory aids. Such an approach, we hope, will also have an impact on the design of prostheses for sufferers of such afflictions as: vocal cord paralysis, spastic dysphonia, glossectomy, pathological pitch deviations, inadequate esophageal speech, and other congenital or traumatic laryngeal deficiencies.

Our modeling studies of coupling characteristics of intraoral acoustic transducers could lead to standards by which future proposed schemes for intraoral speech aids might be evaluated. Specifically, our models and data should make it possible to predict the acoustic performance attainable with any suggested transducer and sensor location. Surgical hazards and other difficulties associated with specific implantation procedures or prostheses could then be weighed in the light of such expected performance.

Information to be gathered on breath control should find application in the design of mobility and communication aids for quadriplegics.

The airflow sensor on the stoma, when developed, may find applications for monitoring the breathing of patients in intensive care units after tracheostomy, following the removal of an artificial respirator. In a modified form it may prove useful in the measurement of airflow during normal speech or singing and, as indicated before, for airflow control by the severely disabled.

Data to be collected on the relationship between f_0 and intensity could lead to some economy in channel-capacity requirements in analysis-synthesis systems in which these are transmitted independently.

REFERENCES

Fant, G.: *Acoustic Theory of Speech Production.* Atlantic Highlands, New Jersey: Mouton and Co., 1960.

Flanagan, J.L.: *Speech Analysis, Synthesis and Perception.* New York: Springer 1972.

Jassem, W.: Normalization of f_0 curves. In Fant, G., and Tatham, M.A.A. (Eds.): *Auditory Analysis and Perception of Speech.* New York: Acad Pr, 1975.

Juang, F., and Markel, J.D.: "Cepstrally based pitch and voicing estimation with statistical assistance." NSC Note No. 140, Signal Technology, Inc., Santa Barbara, California, 1979.

Knorr, S.R., and Zwitman, D.H.: The design of a wireless-controlled intra-oral electrolarynx. *J Bioengineering, 1*:161-171, 1977.

Lieberman, P.: *Intonation, Perception and Language.* Cambridge, MIT Pr, 1967.

Markel, J.D., and Gray, A.H., Jr.: *Linear Prediction of Speech.* New York: Springer, 1976.

Sekey, A.: "Analog Control by Breath Signals." Proceedings Fifth Annual Conference on Systems and Devices for the Disabled. Houston, Texas, June 1978*a*.

———: "Lateral Excitation of a Vocal Tract Analog." Ninth Meeting of the Acoustical Society of America, Honolulu, Hawaii, December 1978*b*.

———: "Towards a Speech Support System for Laryngectomees." Research proposal, 1980.

Sekey, A. and Seagrave, C.: Bidirectional subminiature thermistor sensor for analog control by breath flow. *Biomaterials, Medical Devices and Artificial Organs, 9(1)*:73-90, 1981.

Titze, I.R.: The human vocal cords: a mathematical model. *Phonetica, 28*: 129-170, 1973, and *29*:1-21, 1974.

Weinberg, B., Horii, Y., and Smith, B.E.: Long-time spectral and intensity characteristics of esophageal speech. *J Acoust Soc Am, 67*(5), pp. 1781-4, May, 1980.

Zwitman, D.H., and Disinger, R.S.: Experimental modification of the Western Electric #5 Electrolarynx to a mouth-type instrument. *J Speech Hear Disord, 40*(1): 35-39, 1975.

Zwitman, D.H., Knorr, S., and Sonderman, J.C.: Development and testing of an intra-oral electrolarynx for laryngectomee patients. *J Speech Hear Disord, 43*(2):263-269, 1978.

Chapter 8

THE "INTONATOR": DEVELOPMENT OF AN ELECTROLARYNX WITH INTONATION CONTROL

KAROLY GALYAS, PETER BRANDERUD, AND ROBERT McALLISTER

ABSTRACT

An artificial larynx has been constructed. It has been designed to improve speech naturalness. Continuous control of frequency variation and thus intonation is the most important feature relevant to speech naturalness in this new device. A new design of hardware components makes possible easy handling and increased discretion. These movements have been, in part, motivated by needs expressed by speech therapists and patients. The hardware is composed of three separate components: a vibrator unit, a hand-held control unit, and a power supply/electronics unit. The characteristics of these components are described. Tests and experiments carried out during the development of this device were of two types. One type was concerned with the establishment of optimal electronic and mechanical functions for a group of users. The other type was experiments on the nature of the linguistic relearning task and the facility of learning to speak with this new larynx.

OUR WORK WITH THE development of this new larynx prosthesis was influenced chiefly by the needs of laryngectomized patients and the inability of currently available vibrators to fulfill these needs. We know that many patients make use of electrolarynges, although relatively few are dependent on them as their only voice source. Several surveys show that more than 50 percent of laryngectomees do not develop an acceptable esophageal voice. King, Fowlks, and Pierson (1968) found a figure of 57.4 percent. It is important to the patients that the device be easy to handle and small so as to attract as little attention as possible. An important factor here is, of course, the naturalness of the speech produced with the aid.

An artificial larynx called the *Intonator* was designed with these considerations in mind. The apparatus (*see* Figure 8-1) constructed at the Department of Speech Communication of the Royal Institute of Technology is composed of a small and unobtrusive vibrator unit, a hand-control unit, which can control the frequency and amplitude of the vibration, and a box housing the rechargeable batteries and electronic parts.

The choice of a separate vibrator unit was motivated by demands from laryngectomees. It is an intricate design task to achieve high efficiency with reasonable weight and effective shielding of the directly radiated sound. The present vibrator prototypes utilize the principle of a moving coil connected to a pin that hits the vibrator plate: this arrangement facilitates an efficient energy transfer. The separate vibrator unit is fastened to the neck by means of an elastic band. In the hand-control unit, onset switch and pitch control are separated, permitting an easy

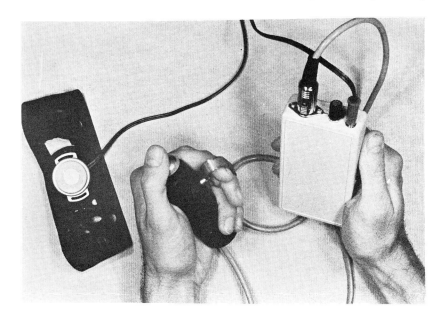

Figure 8-1. The "Intonator" device.

way of obtaining base line frequency as soon as the voice starts. This base line frequency can be individually set, and the pitch can then be varied both above and below this frequency. According to ergonomic studies by Burke and Gibbs (1965), control by force is superior to free movement. This is achieved by spring loading of the pitch-control handle, which limits the maximum displacement to 2 mm.

The small movements are sensed by Hall-effect sensors; the on/off button is operated by the thumb. It is not only a switch function, but there is also a volume control, and, by changing the pressure, the voice intensity can be varied. By means of a volume button the rate of intensity change to pressure variations can be set. Variation of the pitch frequency around the neutral pitch tone is carried out by two other fingers. Squeezing the handle raises the pitch; pulling it out results in a decrease of the pitch frequency. Also incorporated is the possibility to vary the neutral level of pitch frequency and the sensitivity of the pitch control, in order to adapt the aid to the individual user's personal needs.

A series of experiments was undertaken with this new device. The goal of this experimental work was to assess the utility of newly designed electrolarynx and to initiate the development of learning strategies for the use of this new aid. Of particular interest in these experiments was the ability of laryngectomized patients to learn to use the pitch control feature of the Intonator and thereby facilitate more natural speech.

The first experiments were done with a laboratory model; later, take-home prototypes were developed; and finally, three body-worn devices were built for further experiments. The goal of the first series of experiments was to test whether or not the Intonator could be used to produce pitch characteristics of Swedish word accent. There are a number of Swedish word pairs that can be solely distinguished by pitch contour (*see* Gårding, Bruce, and Bannert 1978). Normal subjects were trained in the use of the voice-frequency modulation characteristics. Their tasks included production of simple rises and falls in intonation, as well as the approximation of simple word tone, phrase, and sentence-intonation patterns. The phrases were constructed to give four different meanings, mainly by changing the intonation.

The development of subjects' ability to realize the distinctive Swedish word tones and phrase intonation with the vibrator is seen in Figure 8-2. These are the results of listening tests in which material recorded after each training session was used. Nine listeners were presented with randomly ordered series of stimuli. The test stimuli were composed of pairs of words and pairs of phonetically identical words in all but pitch contour. These minimal pairs were randomly ordered, and the listeners were required to identify the stimuli. After training totalling three hours, the subjects showed reasonable mastery of distinctive pitch contour.

In the second series of experiments, laryngectomized patients

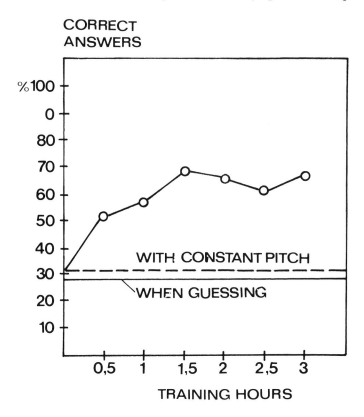

Figure 8-2. Listening tests on word and phrase accent produced by four nonlaryngectomized subjects.

were presented with intonational tasks of varying difficulty similar to the material used in the initial experimental series. They were trained in half-hour sessions, and their progress was carefully recorded. These recordings were the basis of the listening tests that were the same as for the normals in the first series of experiments (20 listeners). Figure 8-3 shows the laryngectomized subjects' progress in the training. One of the subjects had to discontinue the experiments after 3 hours for reasons of health; another one reached 100 percent mastering of the tasks after 3.5 hours of training. A comparison between Figure 8-2 and Figure 8-3 shows clearly the superior performance of the laryngectomized subjects both with constant pitch and with intonation. Subject 1 reaches in fact higher scores with constant pitch than normal subjects with intonation. Being an experienced electrolarynx

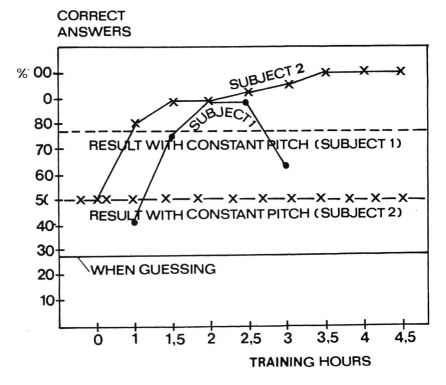

Figure 8-3. Listening tests on word and phrase accent produced by two laryngectomized subjects.

user, he had learned to utilize other prosodic features than just intonation. These results indicate clearly that both normals and laryngectomees can be successful in learning to use this device. These patients, then, have acquired access to a linguistic feature of great importance, not only for linguistic intelligibility but also for emotional expressions.

While the degree of success for the patients was partly dependent on age and emotional adjustment to their handicap, our work indicates that there is a group of laryngectomized individuals whose speech quality could be improved in terms of naturalness and intelligibility through the use of the Intonator.

We are now continuing our work with the refinement of the instrumentation as well as instructional programs to facilitate learning of the important prosodic-control features.

REFERENCES

Burke, D., and Gibbs, C.B.: A comparison of freemoving and pressure levers in a positional control system. *Ergonomics, 8*:23, 1965.

Gårding, E., Bruce, G., and Bannert, R. (Eds.): *Nordic Prosody*, pp. 85-102, Dept. of Linguistics, University of Lund.

King, P.S., Fowlks, E.W., and Pierson, C.A.: Rehabilitation and adaptation of laryngectomy patients. *Am J Phys Med, 47*:192-302, 1968.

Chapter 9

SEMI-AUTOMATIC PITCH CONTROL
FOR AN ELECTROLARYNX

Rob C. van Geel

ABSTRACT

In Dutch intonation, about 70 percent of all pitch contours are variations of the so-called *hat pattern*. The hat pattern is characterized by a fast rise and fall of the fundamental frequency on two accented syllables; furthermore, there is a slow decline in pitch during phonation. This phenomenon is called *declination* and is present in all pitch contours in many languages. A pitch-control circuit for an electrolarynx is described that features these pitch movements, including an automatic declination funtion. A level approach is used in which the transition from a low to a high level constitutes the *fast rise*, and the transition from the high to the low level constitutes the *fast fall*. The advantage of discrete pitch control over continuously variable pitch control is that the excursion and the duration of the pitch movements need not be controlled by the electrolarynx user, and that the control task is limited to the correct placement of the pitch movements in time, in order to induce the perception of sentence accents.

INTRODUCTION

SPEECH PRODUCED WITH AN electrolarynx is monotonous more often than not, even when a device is used which features a pitch control that is not of the preset type (*see* paper by A.W. Knox on "Considerations Toward The Design Of A Totally Automatic Artificial Larynx" in Appendix; also Chap. 6). Apparently electrolarynx users are not able to produce systematic

This research was supported by a grant from the Netherlands Organization for the Advancement of Pure Research (Z.W.O.).

190

pitch variations in their speech. It seems that controlling continuous pitch movements by hand while speaking is too complex. It was thought that a semi-automatic pitch control circuit with which discrete pitch movements can be made would alleviate this complex task. By necessity, such a circuit must incorporate general characteristics of frequent pitch movements.

Considering the availability of Dutch subjects and the fact that the intonation of Dutch is a well-explored subject, the decision was made to base the design of the circuit on Dutch, as far as language-specific features were concerned.

PITCH MOVEMENTS

In research on Dutch intonation, a method has been used that is called *perceptual analysis and resynthesis* (Cohen and 't Hart 1967). In this method, pitch curves were stylized into contours of connecting straight lines. For resynthesis, the original speech signal without its fundamental frequency was used together with the stylized pitch contours. If the pitch contours in the resynthesized speech were judged by a listening panel of Dutch native speakers as perceptually equivalent to those in the original speech samples, the stylizations were used for further analysis. For an extensive description of this method and its application to British English intonation, see De Pijper (1979).

The patterns found in these stylizations appeared to be dependent on a number of discrete pitch movements. Thus, in this approach, intonation is considered to be a dynamic phenomenon, contrary to generally accepted theories of Wells (1945), Pike (1945), and Trager and Smith (1951), who think of intonation as characterized by a sequence of different levels.

From research on Dutch intonation, an inventory has evolved of observed pitch patterns (cf. Collier 1972; 't Hart and Cohen 1973; 't Hart and Collier 1975) of which some main features are discussed here.The main observation in the analysis of the stylized pitch contours was that all contours seem to be tilted. This is called *declination*; it seems to be a phonetic universal (Bolinger 1964; Pierrehumbert 1979; Sorensen and Cooper 1980). Declination is considered to be the result of the decreasing subglottal air pressure during phonation (Collier 1975). Declination is perceptually relevant; an experiment in which the declination line was replaced by a monotonous baseline (Collier 1972) showed that the sentences with the monotonous baseline were judged less natural by a listening panel. Pierrehumbert found that in the perception of, for instance, two tones of different pitch, listeners normalize for expected declination when asked to indicate which tone was higher.

Looking at the patterns found in the stylizations it appeared that the most frequent pattern was the "hat pattern," which, in terms of discrete pitch movements, is characterized by a fast rise and a fast fall on two different syllables. Furthermore, it appeared that many other frequent patterns were variations of the hat pattern. In fact, 70 percent of all Dutch sentences contain these variations (percentage calculated from data in Collier 1972). For the hat pattern and some of its variations, see Figure 9-1.

The excursion of a naturally produced rise or fall is normally limited to about four semitones (1 ST = 1/12 of an octave). This applies also to types of pitch movements other than the fast rise and the fast fall.

In summary, Dutch pitch patterns can be represented by a succession of transitions from the (lower) declination level to a parallel higher level and v.v., with interconnecting stretches along either of these levels ('t Hart 1966).

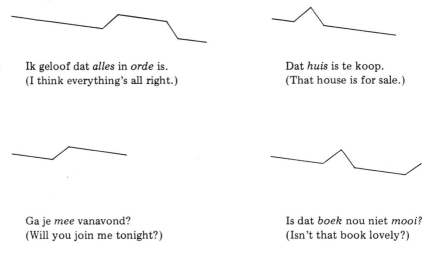

Ik geloof dat *alles* in *orde* is.
(I think everything's all right.)

Dat *huis* is te koop.
(That house is for sale.)

Ga je *mee* vanavond?
(Will you join me tonight?)

Is dat *boek* nou niet *mooi?*
(Isn't that book lovely?)

Figure 9-1. Examples of the Dutch hat pattern and the variants.

PITCH CONTROL CIRCUIT

It was decided to build-in an automatic declination function in the control circuit, as absence of declination is one of the causes of the unnaturalness of the monotonous quality of average electrolarynx speech. In speech synthesis, declination is usually set at a value of about -2 ST/sec for short sentences up to 4 seconds.* Specifying in semitones has the advantage that, as the semitone is a logarithmic unit, the absolute frequency levels off in time, so that pitch does not drop unnaturally low.

Furthermore, the fast rise and the fast fall were included in the control circuit. For the fast rise, an average increase in pitch of 4 ST in 100 msec has been observed and, for the fast fall, an average decrease in pitch of -5 ST in 150 msec ('t Hart and Cohen 1973). For reasons of simplicity in the circuit design, however, the fast fall was specified as a decrease in pitch of -4 ST in 100 msec. In this way it was possible to utilize a second level, parallel to the declination level, which is 4 ST higher. The desired pitch movements can be made by electronic control of the transition time from one level to the other.

The pitch movements are made in the following way: the lower declination is started when a control button on the electrolarynx is depressed. When the control is slid forward a resistor in the declination generator is short-circuited, which causes the pitch of the oscillation circuit driving the vibrator of the electrolarynx to follow the upper declination level (*see* Figure 9-2). Pitch drops back to the lower declination level when the control is moved backward again (*see* Figure 9-3). Releasing the control either in the lower or upper declination level position causes the output to be switched off and the declination to be reset in silence at the beginning of the low declination level. This was done deliberately, as most Dutch sentences start at the lower declination level. For an example of a simple hat contour produced with the electrolarynx prototype, which is controlled by the previously mentioned circuit (*see* Figure 9-4). As can be seen in this registration, the pitch starts at ca. 100 Hz and drops gradually when the device is switched on. For the time being, attention has been focused on

---

*J.R. De Pijper: personal communication.

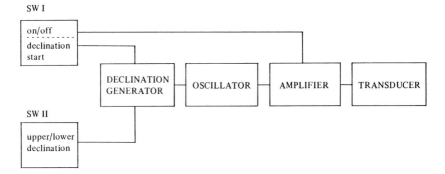

Figure 9-2. Block diagram of the pitch-control circuit including switches.

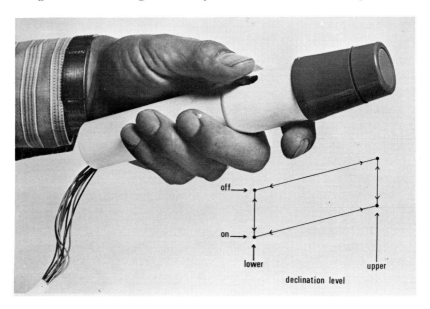

Figure 9-3. Electrolarynx prototype and diagram of the movements of the pitch-control button.

the pitch-control principle. The duration of the fast rise, however, does not yet conform to the specifications given, and no attempt has been made to optimize actual output volume, although quite acceptable results are obtained by utilizing an existing transducer (by Servox) and by driving it with a sawtooth wave.

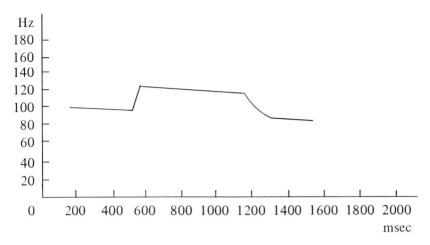

Figure 9-4. Hat contour made with the electrolarynx prototype.

SUMMARY

There is one aspect that should be mentioned first, as it is the main reason for the failure of electrolarynx speakers to adequately control the pitch of their electrolarynx: they are not conscious of *what pitch is* and *which pitch movements and patterns are possible* in their language. To fill in this gap, separate training sessions in post-laryngectomy rehabilitation in the use and control of pitch are required. This is important, irrespective of the type of pitch variation on the electrolarynx used—continuous or discrete—excluding, of course those electrolarynges that only feature a preset pitch control. Conscious knowledge of native pitch patterns is a necessary condition for adequate use of the possibilities of the electrolarynx.

The advantage of this electrolarynx prototype over one which features continuous pitch control can be explained as follows. As mentioned previously, the excursion of pitch movements is limited, as is the case in any language. Furthermore, it is easy to see that it is simpler to effect a rise or a fall in a pitch contour than to effect a rise or a fall, and at the same time a gradual fall (= declination), throughout the utterance. In other words, the task of the electrolarynx user is simpler when the only thing that has to be taken care of in pitch control is the correct placement of the pitch movements on the syllables to be accented.

Although the electrolarynx described here is based on Dutch intonation, it must be stressed that the main underlying principle, namely, the automatic declination function, is applicable to many other languages as well. In fact, with the device as it is, it is possible to produce some British-English sentences in which there are pitch movements similar to the Dutch ones used. Some examples, based on observed pitch contours, are given in Figure 9-5 (declination is omitted for graphical reasons).

The use of discrete pitch movements in electrolarynx speech is limited to languages in which the most frequent pitch patterns can be made with a small subset of pitch movements, because the more pitch movements that are necessary, the more difficult becomes its control. In Dutch, it is not only possible to produce about 70 percent of all observed pitch patterns with a subset of two pitch movements, but it is also perfectly natural to the casual Dutch listener if only speech with variations of the hat pattern is used (Collier and 't Hart 1977).

Automatic declination can be used in almost any language. It may even be combined with continuous pitch control in which pitch movements can be superimposed on the declination.

A discrete pitch control with fixed pitch movements has the additional advantage that the user need not concern himself with the excursion and duration of the pitch movements.

To summarize, the three difficult factors in controlling the pitch of an electrolarynx, that is, declination, type of pitch

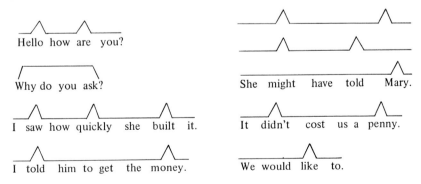

Figure 9-5. Examples of British-English sentences with pitch movements similar to Dutch.

movement, and placement of pitch movement, have been reduced to the last factor only. Under these conditions, only limited knowledge of intonation phenomena is necessary for the user of an electrolarynx based on the previously mentioned principles.

REFERENCES

Bolinger, D.: Intonation as a universal. *Proc. IXth Int. Congr. Linguists*: 833. The Hague: Mouton, 1964.

Cohen, A., and 't Hart, J.: On the anatomy of intonation. *Lingua, 19*: 177, 1967.

Collier, R.: *From Pitch to Intonation*. Dissertation Leuven, Belgium, 1972.

————: Physiological correlates of intonation. *JASA, 58*: 249, 1975.

Collier, R., and 't Hart, J.: *Cursus Nederlandse Intonatie*. W.O.L., Belgium: Diepenbeek, 1977.

De Pijper, J.R.: Close copy stylizations of British English intonation contours. *IPO Annual Progress Report, 14*:66, 1979.

Pierrehumbert, J.: The perception of fundamental frequency declination. *JASA, 66*:363, 1979.

Pike, K.L.: *The intonation of American English*. Ann Arbor: U of Mich Pr, 1945.

Sorensen, J.M., and Cooper, W.E.: Syntactic coding of fundamental frequency in speech production. In Cole, R.A. (Ed.): *Perception and Production of Fluent Speech*. Hillsdale, N.J.: Lawrence Erlbaum, 1980.

't Hart, J.: Perceptual analysis of Dutch intonation features. *IPO Annual Progress Report, 1*:47, 1966.

't Hart, J., and Cohen, A.: Intonation by rule: a perceptual quest. *J Phonetics 1*: 309, 1973.

't Hart, J., and Collier, R.: Integrating different levels of intonation analysis. *J Phonetics 3*:235, 1975.

Trager, G.L., and Smith, H.L.: An outline of English structure. *Studies in Linguistics Occ. Papers 3*. Norman, Battenburg Press, 1951.

Wells, R.: The pitch phonemes of English. *Language, 21*:27, 1945.

Chapter 10

AN ARTIFICIAL VOICING WAVEFORM
FOR LARYNGECTOMEES

J. Bach Andersen, B. Langvad, H. Møller, and O. Rold

ABSTRACT

The well-known mechanical artificial larynx is placed externally against the lower throat and excites, through vibrations, the vocal-tract resonances. Not all laryngectomees are able to use this aid and for patients in intensive care it may be impossible. A compact speech aid consisting of a portable sound generator and a thin plastic tube has been developed. A periodic signal, stored in a memory, excites a small loudspeaker, which again excites the tube. The tube is placed in the back of the mouth. The device is in principle similar to earlier mechanical devices. The new idea involves the possibility of optimizing the waveform for maximum intelligibility, partly compensating for the nonoptimized position of the source. For maximum power output, tube resonances are utilized. In developing the waveform, speech tests and spectrograph analysis have been used.

BACKGROUND

THE MOST-USED SPEECH aid for persons without a larynx is the mechanical vibrator, which is externally pressed against the neck tissues. There are several situations where this device is difficult to use. One of these is in the case of older people, where the transmission through the flesh impairs

Mr. Niels Pedersen is gratefully acknowledged for the practical construction of the prototype, the phonetics laboratory of Arhus University for the loan of their spectrograph, and the ENT department of Aalborg Hospital South for their support. The work was supported by Aalborg City's Foundation for Medical Research.

an efficient coupling to the oral cavities. Another is the situation in the hospital, where patients in intensive care have temporarily lost the use of their larynx and are unable to use a mechanical device. In the latter situation there is an urgent need for communication, which requires a simple apparatus to be used without extensive training.

The device to be described rests on the simple idea of putting an external sound source into the mouth to replace the lost larynx or, for patients in intensive care, the blocked larynx. Since the remainder of the person's articulatory system is intact, he just "speaks" as usual as if he had a larynx. Earlier versions of this device exist, e.g. in the form of a pipe with a small mechanical vibrator in the pipe head. This new version relies on modern electronic circuitry, which makes it relatively easy to create various spectral distributions and various pitch heights.

In the following, the design of the apparatus is described in detail, and some results and performance tests are discussed.

DESCRIPTION OF APPARATUS

A photo of a prototype version is shown in Figure 10-1 and in a block diagram in Figure 10-2. The system generates a periodic

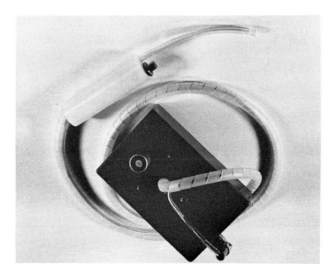

Figure 10-1. Photograph of prototype voice generator.

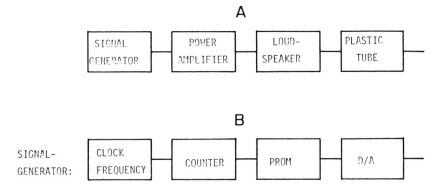

Figure 10-2. (*A*) Block diagram of the system; and (*B*) signal-generating system.

signal with a time period corresponding to a pitch of 120 Hz for men and 240 Hz for women. The time sequence within a period is stored in a PROM as indicated; the time variation of the signal will be discussed later. After a digital-to-analogue conversion, a power amplifier excites a small loudspeaker, which again excites a 1.5 m long plastic tube. A periodic sound signal with a prescribed power spectrum is emitted from the end of the tube, which is put into the mouth. The diameter of the tube is only about 5 mm, and it creates only minor articulation problems to have the tube in the mouth. A small switch in the hand turns the power on or off, but the pitch and level of the signal are constant.

THE ACOUSTICAL SYSTEM

Two design criteria are important for the acoustical system, by which we mean the loudspeaker and tube. The system must be power efficient, since we are using a battery-driven energy source, and it must be able to cover the necessary frequency range. The system and its electrical analogue are shown in Figure 10-3, where the tube is modelled by a transmission line. It is important that the loudspeaker be shielded, since a direct "unmodulated" signal from the box will have a deteriorating effect on the intelligibility of speech. One of the problems with the mechanical vibrator is that the articulated sound must compete with the direct signal from the vibrator.

Analysis of the system shows that the tube resonances can be used advantageously since we have a periodic source. The lowest frequency (120 Hz for men) corresponds to a tube length of 1.50 m for half a wavelength. The details of the analysis are not given here; however, the conclusions derived from data analysis are that the membrane area should be small in order to give a high-resonance frequency. Furthermore, the $B \times 1$ product of the loudspeaker should be high. Figure 10-3C shows the transfer function of the system from the voltage input to received sound pressure 10 cm from the tube ending.

Although the impedance of the load changes when the tube is in the mouth, analysis and experience show that the mismatch from the generator to the load is so large that we can assume that the flow at the tube ending is effectively independent of acoustical loading, i.e. independent of the position in the mouth.

THE ELECTRICAL SYSTEM

The electrical system gives the input to the loudspeaker as previously described, the critical point being the shape of the signal. If we know the required spectrum at the tube ending, it is a simple matter to find the electrical signal as a function of time. The problem is, of course, that the complete system includes the oral cavities of the patient, taking into account that the source is displaced relative to the natural position of the larynx.
larynx.

The first attempt to find the optimum spectrum is based on the philosophy that the vowels should be correct on average, since they are the main components depending on the spectrum of the vocal cords.

The spectrum has been found by a substitution method, where

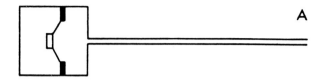

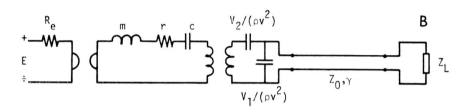

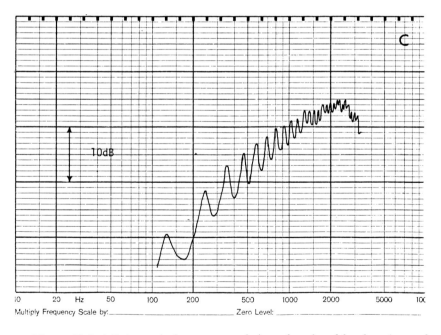

Figure 10-3. (*A*) Acoustical system consisting of enclosed loudspeaker and tube; (*B*) electrical equivalent circuit of (*A*); and (*C*) sound pressure measured 10 cm in front of tube ending for constant voltage input.

a normal speaker pronounces a vowel with his natural voice and afterwards makes an effort to do the same with the tube in the mouth and a known electrical-input spectrum. The difference spectrum was averaged over all vowels and over four speakers; the power spectrum of the input signal could then be determined.

Utilizing the fact that the ear is insensitive to phase, the phases of the various harmonics may be shuffled around to give a minimum peak-to-peak signal, which is significant for an efficient use of the battery voltage. The resulting signal shape in the time domain was found by using an optimization technique; an example for the male voice is shown in Figure 10-4. In this system, 256 different points of the period are stored with an eight-bit accuracy in the memory.

PERFORMANCE

In its present form the speech aid is not fully satisfactory. It has been used successfully by some volunteers, but it seems to require a little training. Especially for patients in bed it has been difficult in the sense that the intelligibility was low, perhaps because the original spectrum was developed with the aid of healthy subjects who simulated a closed glottis.

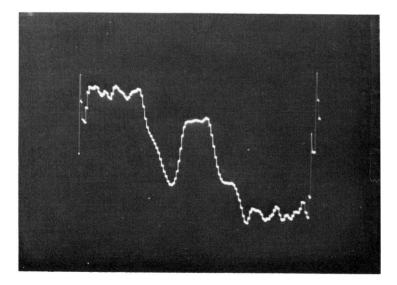

Figure 10-4. One period of electrical input to loudspeaker.

In Figure 10-5, spectrograms are shown of a Danish sentence spoken by one of the authors with (*a*) a natural voice, (*b*) a speech aid and closed glottis, and (*c*) a speech aid, open glottis, and open to the nasal cavity. It is clear that the situation in (*c*) is considerably worse than in (*b*).

Comparing Figure 10-5*a* and 10-5*b*, it is noted that smooth formant transitions in natural speech are only partly reconstructed. One explanation for this may be that the position of the sound inside the cavity instead of at one end introduces zeros in the transfer function at certain frequencies. These zeros may not be fully compensated with the chosen signal due to the narrow bandwidth of the zeros. One possible remedy for this may be a multielement source.

$\longrightarrow$

Figure 10-5. The Danish sentence "Laila bor i lejlighed" spoken by one of the authors: (*A*) with natural voice; (*B*) with speech aid and closed glottis; and (*C*) with speech aid and glottis open to nasal cavity.

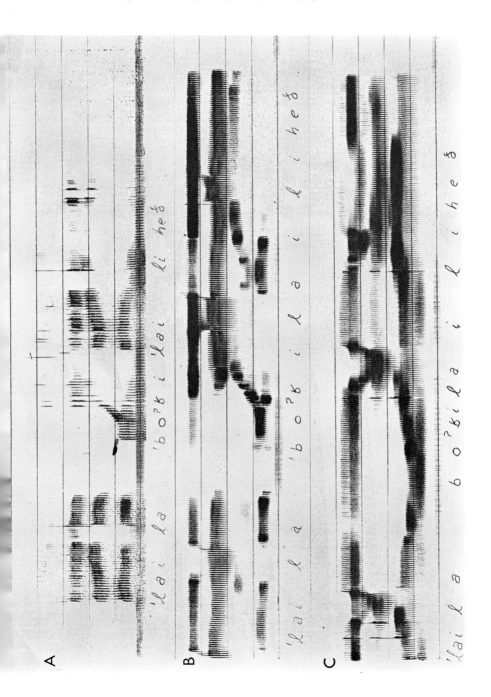

ON OBJECTIVE TESTING
OF SPEECH AMPLIFIERS

KAROLY GALYAS AND PETER BRANDERUD

ABSTRACT

A number of acoustical and electrical parameters are defined, and their significance in practical performance of speech amplifiers is discussed as follows:

a. Highest useful amplification, measured at a volume-control setting below the level of acoustic feedback ("howling")
b. Highest useful speech output level with acceptable quality
c. Frequency response
d. Distortion, measured at different sound levels and frequencies
e. Sound level when howling
f. Noise level
g. Power consumption when quiet and at a specified sound level

Methods used for measuring the above parameters are described, and some results and recommendations are presented. The results of the objective measurements correspond well with the patients' subjective judgments. Described methods are suggested to be used as a basis for establishing international norms.

P ERSONS WITH WEAK voices often experience the frustration of not being able to make themselves heard in noisy environments. This problem can be overcome through the use of some kind of amplification. There are many different aids and devices offered to the handicapped, from large public-address systems to small speech amplifiers with varying quality and usefulness.

It is reasonable to require this kind of aid to provide a sufficient and good quality amplification of the user's speech, to keep the risk for acoustic feedback at a minimum, to be easy for the user to carry and to put into operation, and to be economical.

It is hard to fulfill all the above requirements, and there are a number of compromises taken in this kind of aid. Amplifiers available on the market perform differently due to emphasis on different features. There is a need for objective testing methods to facilitate comparison of different technical solutions. On a contract from the Swedish Institute for the Handicapped, we worked out methods for measuring a number of electroacoustic parameters and tested five available amplifiers. A detailed description of the measurement methods and results are published in Swedish in a technical report from the Department of Speech Communication (*see* Branderud 1976). The same devices were also subjectively evaluated by two logopedists, Bergström and Stendahl (1973). The main purpose here is to describe the measurement methods, give some results, and discuss requirements; the results are put together in Table 11-I. The amplifiers measured are listed next. The results should not be used to form opinions on currently available amplifiers due to the fact that all devices tested were produced before 1974.

1. An industrial prototype of the Speech Amplifier TF-2, produced by Special Instrument AB. Size 150 × 67 × 24 mm. Microphone electret, directivity type. Battery 9.6v rechargeable type.

2. Development prototype from Norway. Size 94 × 70 × 30 mm. Microphone dynamic, omnidirectional type. Battery 9v standard.

3. *Emitron®*, produced by Sama, Italy. Size 80 × 80 × 30 mm. Microphone dynamic, omnidirectional type. Battery 8.5v rechargeable type.

4. S.G. Brown Therapeutic Speech Amplifier, produced by S.G. Brown Ltd., Great Britain. Size 105 × 63 × 27 mm. Microphone dynamic, omnidirectional type, throat microphone and lightweight headset available. Battery 9v standard type.

5. *CommunicAid®*, produced by A.R. Mann, USA. Size

89 × 63 × 31 mm. Microphone dynamic, omnidirectional type. Battery 9v standard type.

ELECTRICAL AND ACOUSTICAL MEASUREMENTS

In the following measurements the amplifier is always in a breast pocket of a person, 25 cm from the mouth to simulate the natural situation.

Highest Useful Amplification

The most important parameter is the maximum possible amplification. Because of the small distance between the microphone and loudspeaker, this will be limited by the acoustical feedback in the system.

With the microphone 0.5 cm in front of the mouth and the amplifier in the breast pocket, the volume setting was adjusted to be as high as possible without howling feedback noise. The setting must allow minor movements of the microphone without howling because of reflected sound waves. This setting was then used in the measurements.

When measuring the amplification, a B & K type 4219 artificial mouth with an opening of 20 mm was used. It was fed with white noise filtered in such a way that the output from the mouth had the same average spectrum as male speech, measured by Fletcher (1953) (cf. Figure 11-1). The mouth is first compensated to give a flat response and the spectrum can then be approximated by the circuit in Figure 11-2. The use of this voice source reduced the measurement time considerably and made the measurements repeatable.

The data in Table 11-1 show the difference in sound level with and without amplification—defined as the difference between sound levels with the amplifier switched on and off—measured at a distance of 1 m from both the microphone and the loudspeaker (cf. Figure 11-3). There were considerable differences between the amplifiers. The value of this important parameter is dependent on the directivity of the microphone and the resonances in the frequency response of the system. The outstanding performance of amplifier No. 1 results mainly from the small

Table 11-I

Results		1	2	3	4	5
				Speech Amplifier No.		
A. Highest useful amplification	(dB)	29	19	19	21 15 (a)	17
B. Highest useful speech sound level at a distance of 1 m	(dB)	73	66	65	59	64
C. Distortion (%) at levels −3, −10, −20 dB below clipping level and at frequencies 500, 1000, and 2000 Hz,	−3 dB	3.0 2.0 1.4	18 7 7	2.0 1.2 1.0	14 20 2.0	20 3.3 8
	−10 dB	2.5 1.0 0.8	13 5 3	4.0 2.0 1.5	23 12 1.0	18 1.2 7
	−20 dB	0.7 1.5 0.3	45 4 1	1.0 0.5 0.6	7 9 0.7	25 5.0 6
E. Sound level when howling (dist. 1 m)	(dB SPL)	65	92	85	75	88
F. Noise level at a distance of 1 m.	(dB SPL)	13 (b)	36	18 (b)	18 (b)	7
G1. Power consumption at a sound level of 66 dB SPL (distance 1 m).	(mW)	130	175	170	115	80
G2. Power consumption when idle.	(mW)	33	135	135	70	30
H1. Calculated operation time at a sound level of 66 dB SPL 50% of time.	(hours)	28	4.0	12	5.5	8
H2. Calculated operation time when idle	(hours)	70	4.7	15	9	21

Remarks (a) when using headset microphone
(b) noise level is proportional to volume setting

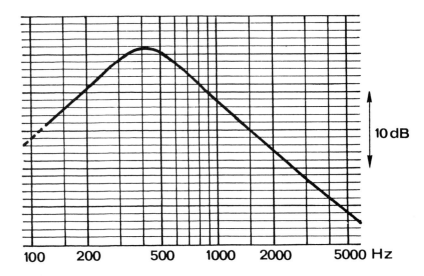

Figure 11-1. Average spectrum of male speech.

differential microphone, which can be placed very near the mouth. Finally, the highest useful amplification should be as high as possible: the higher, the better.

Highest Useful Speech Sound Level At a Distance Of 1 Meter With Acceptable Sound Quality

Clipping of the signal at high levels results in high distortion, which is not acceptable. The highest useful speech sound level with acceptable sound quality is defined as the highest average level of speech with acceptable distortion of the peak signals. When measuring this, the same sound source as above was used.

The noise level was raised until the output from the loud-speaker was considerably distorted. The absolute, dominating part of the distortion in a good amplifier comes from the clipping in the electronic circuit.

To get a well-defined distortion, the noise should be increased until the "difference" between the levels on meter 2 and meter 1 has been reduced by 3 db. The reading of meter 2 must be lowered by 10 db to get the value at 1 m instead of 30 cm (*see* Figure 11-4).

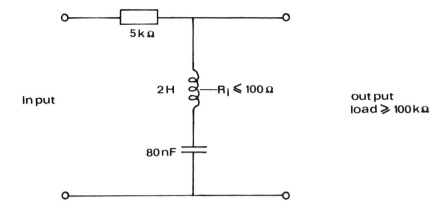

Figure 11-2. Filter for approximating spectrum in Figure 11-1 from white noise.

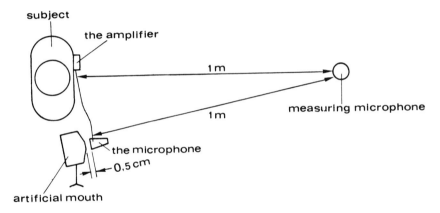

Figure 11-3. Setup for measuring amplification.

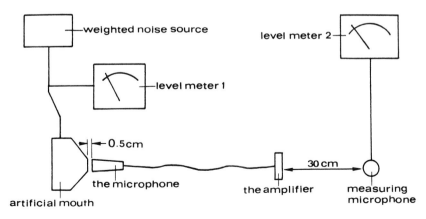

Figure 11-4. Setup for measuring the highest useful speech sound level.

This sound level is proportional to some mean values of the clipping levels at different frequencies. Sixteen db was subtracted from this level. The value of 16 db is the result of listening tests of acceptable distortion.

Even if the value 16 db could be disputed, the method gives a tool to compare different amplifiers and an idea about the highest acceptable quality speech sound level at a distance of 1 m from each amplifier.

The values in the Table 11-I can be compared to a normal speech level, which is around 66 db SPL. In noisy environments it is often much higher. A 6-db difference between two amplifiers makes quite a big difference. This parameter again should be as high as possible.

In some situations a very bad quality could be accepted, as when crying for help. In such a case a 10-16 db higher sound level can be achieved.

Frequency Response

The frequency response was measured in an anechoic chamber. This measurement can also be made with acceptable results in a normal damped room, if the measuring microphone is placed about 30 cm instead of 1 m in front of the loudspeaker. The distance to a reflecting object should be at least 1-1.5 m. There were big differences between the amplifiers. No. 2 and No. 5 had a bad response (-20 to -10 db) in the range of 300-1000 Hz, and this makes the voice sharp and artificial. Our experience is that most subjects wanted the amplifier to reproduce the speech as natural as possible. The frequency response over the range of 400-4000 Hz should be flat within ± 5 db. A narrow dip of 5-10 db at around 1300 Hz has been observed, which is caused by reflection from the body and can be neglected.

DISTORTION AT DIFFERENT SOUND LEVELS

The distortion was measured by a sinusoidal tone with the frequencies 500 Hz, 1 kHz, and 2kHz. The levels were at -3 db, -10 db, and -20 db relative to the clipping level. Three of the amplifiers had very high distortion at 500 Hz. The distortion makes the voice harsh, sharp, or blurry and it should be held low: 5 percent is probably an acceptable limit.

Sound Level When Howling

It can be very annoying for a user when the amplifier starts to howl. This risk is especially great when the volume control is adjusted or the microphone is moved. The maximum level when howling was measured at a distance of 1m. Normally this value will be high when the value of measurement B is high, though amplifier 1 is an exception. It has an electronic circuit, which gives it a very low howling level.

Noise Level

It is important that the amplifier be "silent" in the silent periods of speech. The A-weighted noise level was measured at a short distance of 1 cm from the amplifier, and the corresponding noise level at a distance of 1 m was calculated by adding 36 db. The same amplification as in measurement A was used. The noise can be disturbing when it is above 20 db in a silent environment. The noise from amplifier 2 was very disturbing.

Power Consumption and Operation Time

It is important to know if the time between battery changes or charging of the accumulator is sufficient for the current user, as the cost for battery use will be important. The power consumption was measured at a speech level of 66 db SPL and when idle. The operation time when speaking 50 percent of the time and the operation time when in idle was also measured.

SUMMARY

The results of the objective measurements correspond well with the patients' subjective judgments of the amplifiers and with their performance in practical situations (*see* Bergström and Stendahl 1973). Therefore, it is hoped that these objective measurements can form a basis for judgment of the utility of these aids by the speech handicapped. In the light of the need for international, objective norms of this nature, we would suggest that the above-described methods could be used as a basis for establishing such standards.

REFERENCES

Bergström, H., and Stendahl, M.: "Funktionell provning av röstapparater och talförstärkare för laryngectomerade," thesis work in logopedics, Department of Logopedics and Phoniatrics, Huddinge Hospital, Karolinska, Huddinge, Sweden, 1973.

Branderud, P.: "Provning av talförstärkare för handikappade med svag röst." Dept. of Speech Communication, KTH, Technical Rep. STL-TR-1976-1, 1976.

Fletcher, H. (1953): *Speech and Hearing in Communication.* Princeton: van Nostrand, 1953.

IMPLANTED ELECTROLARYNGEAL PROSTHESIS

R.L. EVERETT AND B.J. BAILEY

ABSTRACT

A surgically implantable electrolaryngeal prosthesis offers great possibilities in the production of high-quality speech, besides offering great convenience and social acceptability. In this chapter the acoustic difficulties of external prostheses are shown to derive from many acoustic inadequacies, and it is shown that the implant unit has excellent acoustic advantage. The state of the art of electrolaryngeal prostheses is reviewed and current efforts compared. The design parameters of the entire system are reviewed and are shown to be derived from functional necessity. Manners of control of the devices are discussed, and the pulse technique for the synthesis of appropriate vocal-tract vibrations is discussed.

Progress in hardware, surgical technique, and materials is given exposition.

INTRODUCTION

THE DESIRABILITY OF implanted electrolaryngeal prostheses is based largely on their promise of being eventually able to generate high-quality speech, that is, speech having the esthetic qualities of the natural human voice. Besides this promise, the implanted prosthesis should be more convenient and have an increased social acceptability.

Other forms of laryngeal prostheses certainly generate intelligible speech, but equally certainly do not generate high-quality speech. For this reason, and those of inconvenience, low social

---

This work was supported in part by NLI research grant CA17961-01 from the NCI.

acceptability of the (usually) unsightly apparatus and the jarring effect of the speech produced by them, the external prostheses are not widely accepted.

In order to appreciate the excellent prospects of high-quality speech production by implanted electrolaryngeal prostheses, one needs to understand the severe acoustic problems of the external hand-held laryngeal prosthesis.

The stages of speech production by this method start with the production of a vibration, which is mechanically coupled to the anterior cervical tissues, through which the vibrations are transmitted to the interior vocal-tract cavity walls, which in vibrating, couples the vibrations into the vocal-tract air column. From there, normal speech-production processes take over, the various resonances of the vocal-tract shape the harmonic spectrum of the vocal-tract vibrations, and out of the buccal aperture speech may come.

The above sequence of activities appears straightforward and uninvolved. But each stage in the process is subject to various difficulties, and the overall effect can be far from that desired.

To start with, there is an inevitable interaction between the vibration source, usually some sort of electromechanical transducer, and the tissue of the throat. The vibrator puts a force on the tissue and accelerates it. But, in turn, the tissue puts a force on the transducer, and this force degrades the transducer performance. This is a mass-loading effect on the transducer. The overall result is that the acceleration of the transducer is diminished, and the overall deflection of the vibrating surface of the transducer is smaller. So, the effective sound output of the wave coupled into the tissue is smaller in amplitude, and the wave shape produced is modified. Hand-held prostheses are also subject to large variations of application pressure, so that the loading effects are variable in nature. Since the nature of mass-loaded transducers is such that the system forms a low-pass filter in the transmission function from electric signal to sound pressure level (SPL) in the neck tissue, the overall tendency is to smooth the SPL wave shape and reduce sharp-wave components. Such smoothing may or may not be desirable, but its variability introduces serious complications in the formation of quality speech.

Once a sound wave is introduced into the anterior surface of the neck tissue, it must propagate through the neck tissue to the anterior pharyngeal wall. There are in general two effects that complicate this innocent-appearing process.

First, the transducer is usually a quite localized source of sound, which excites a highly localized area of neck tissue. But the neck tissue, even in the most radical of laryngectomies, is a highly nonuniform mass of muscle and membrane. The properties of sound propagation through such an inhomogeneous medium is such that there is much spreading of the sound wave from the localized source. Second, because of mass-spring-viscous damping effects, there is a shift of phase and an amplitude variation of the various harmonics of the impressed wave over the different paths from transducer to pharynx.

These two points are important from the standpoint of speech quality for the following reason: the vocal tract forms a distributed parameter acoustic transmission line, and the output of such a line is different for different application points of the exciting wave. The physical spread of the excitation wave and its amplitude and phase variations excite the vocal tract in a distributed fashion,' and the output wave is the sum of the responses to the aggregate excitation, so that the resultant voice wave is not what would be expected from the given original mechanical oscillation applied to the neck.

It is certainly possible to determine a mechanical wave that would result in excellent speech quality for at least one vowel sound under static throat muscle and tissue conditions. Even if a mechanical excitation wave does indeed exist that gives good speech quality for a given set of vowel sounds for a given throat application position and pressure, a certain element of variability will be introduced by slight positional error in application location of a hand-held prosthesis.

Further variability in the quality of speech produced by a hand-held electrolaryngeal prosthesis is introduced by the variability of mass and tonus of the throat muscles, by tissue degeneration effects such as due to radiation treatment, or by post operative scar tissue buildup.

All of these factors affect, mostly in a negative way, the speech quality of the external electrolaryngeal prosthesis.

Now speech intelligibility of such devices can be enhanced by word-phrase correlated tonal inflection of the oscillation frequency of the applied mechanical vibration. There are a multitude of techniques for effecting such speech modulation; some of these will be discussed in the applicable section on implantable electrolaryngeal prosthesis. It should be pointed out here that many of the factors affecting speech quality in the external prosthesis also make tone modulation difficult. Several of the most critical factors are mass-loading effects on the transducer and all of the variability effects in application position and pressure.

Finally, speech intelligibility in the hand-held electrolaryngeal prosthesis is adversely affected by competition between the two acoustic signals produced by the external vibration source. The desired component, speech, is projected from the mouth. The not-desired "noise" component is that radiated directly from the vibrator and superficial throat. Poorly designed, held, or placed external prostheses have a poor signal-to-noise ratio, wherein the desired intelligible signal is masked by the direct radiated noise component and, therefore, intelligibility suffers.

In spite of these problems with external electrolaryngeal prostheses, there is a great deal that can be done to significantly improve the quality and intelligibility of speech produced by them. Such work deserves immediate priorities because of the immediacy of possible results that could benefit those many laryngectomees who do not benefit from the advantages to be derived from the implantable electrolaryngeal prosthesis.

It is with pleasure that one contemplates the enormous simplification in the acoustical situation of an implanted electrolaryngeal prosthesis, in comparison with that of the external unit. The basic differences are immediately apparent. Given the possibility of surgical implantation, the vocal-tract excitation sound source may be placed at approximately the same location in the pharynx as the natural sound source, the larynx. Since the transducer forms a highly localized vibrational source in the vocal tract, distributed excitation effects and harmonic phase-amplitude effects may be avoided. Tissue-loading effects on the transducer are inherently small, and the mechanical forces acting on the vibrator are stationary or, at worst, very slowly varying. The acoustic radiation component direct from vibrator to auditor should be quite small, being transmitted through neck tissue before reaching an open air-path.

By implanting an electrolaryngeal prosthesis in the appropriate place, one accrues, therefore, great advantages in speech quality and intelligibility over an external prosthesis. The price one pays for these advantages is great. The demands in device reliability and performance are great; the biocompatibility requirements are just now within the state of the art, though there is a risk of infection. Economic considerations cannot be evaluated at this time, although every attempt at arriving at a moderate hardware and surgical procedure cost is being made.

The basic requirements of an implanted electrolaryngeal prosthesis are (1) a vibration source that can cause acoustic waves of the proper amplitude, fundamental frequency, and harmonic content in the vocal tract; (2) a manner of powering this implanted source from outside the body; and (3) on-off keying capability with provisions for pitch inflection and amplitude control.

PRIOR ART

Considering the difficulty of maintaining operative a chronically implanted electromechanical or electronic-electromechanical device, one should not be startled to discover that the history of such efforts is brief.

Many efforts were made that skirted the principal issues of an implanted device. For example, intraoral devices like tooth-shaped sound sources, or dental plate mounted sound sources (Tait 1959) with wireless power transduction are ingenious and interesting. These have a potentially low accident rate because of their accessibility for repair. Unfortunately, speech volume and quality from such devices has been to date unacceptable.

Goode (1969) described a technique that, although utilizing an external electronic sound source, used a pharyngocutaneous fistula for introducing the sound into the proper elevation in the vocal tract. The sound output from such a system may have high intelligibility, but has small potential for high quality because of the severe acoustic tuning effects of a tube of any length.

Besides our own, there is only one other group working on a true electrolaryngeal prosthesis. That group is at the University of Toronto, and their work slightly antedates ours.

The Canadian group reports (Rogers, Frederickson, and Bryce 1975; Griffiths, Frederickson, and Bryce 1976; Frederickson 1980) that they have evolved a linear electromagnetic vibration source with an implant capacity. This device may be implanted at a level about even with the larynx. Power is supplied to it by a subcutaneous pair of wires which terminate on a bipolar connector mounted on a bioCarbon button, which provides a means of through-the-skin electric signal transport. The signal source that drives the transducer is an oscillator with a power amplifier on the output. Tone and voice volume are controlled by a joystick.

The Canadian electrolaryngeal prosthesis underwent sufficient testing in dogs to allow human trial. Two human subjects had the device implanted for about a year each. The voice quality was reported (Frederickson 1980) to be about that of a good Western Electric electrolarynx user; voice volume was adjudged to be adequate.

One device was removed because of a failure due to a broken wire. The other device was removed because projection of the vibration source into the subject's pharynx (which had a compromised lumen due to prior surgery) caused swallowing difficulty and led to substantial weight loss in the patient.

The Canadian development went through a different sequence of activity than did ours. Also, different aspects of the electrolaryngeal prosthesis system were stressed in the development processes. However, it seems that important similarities in thinking and technique exist between the two systems. In the following pages these and some of the interesting differences between the two systems will be noted.

OUR DEVELOPMENTAL APPROACH

Initial investigations into the constraints and practicalities of the implanted electrolaryngeal prosthesis problem were along the following lines.

Anatomical studies of the human neck (and that of a dog, as an experimental animal) revealed that the simplest place to install a vibration source was the *retropharynx* and, for acoustical reasons, at about the level of the fifth cervical vertebra. For purposes of coupling well the vibration through the pharyngeal wall into the vocal-tract air column, the diameter of the vibration source should not be less than the physical extent of the pharyngeal wall it contacts. The thickness of the vibration source should be maximally 1.2 cm, and the thinner the better so as not to seriously occlude the pharyngeal lumen. The mechanical driving capabilities of the transducer should be such that its performance remains essentially unmodified by the need to drive tissue, whose total mass might run as high as 30 gm.

At that time, the decision was also made to use wireless power transmission, rather than risk direct transdermal power connections.

Thus, by implication, the broad outline of the electrolaryngeal prosthesis system was set. It was to be composed of some sort of electromechanical transducer as vibration source, which was powered by some pulsatile electric signal. At this time the configuration of the electromechanical transducer was chosen to be a magnetically biased, nonlinear, magnetically actuated device. This selection was made because of the outstanding electric-to-vibration conversion of this type of device.

Further, it was determined, in order to ease the reliability problem, to have as few electronic components in the subdermal unit as possible. In order to minimize possibility of complication due to infection, a wireless, transdermal, power-transmitting system was to be implemented. Thus, the subdermal unit was to be composed of a subdermal, power-pickup coil, a rectifier-filter unit, and the electromechanical transducer.

The extradermal unit must supply an RF power signal (amplitude modulated in an appropriate fashion) to excite the implant device.

The overall design projection of the Canadian prosthesis is in broad detail very similar to ours. The only significant difference lies in their choice of a hard, through-the-skin, wired power-transmission technique. This eliminated the RF power transmitter, the transformer arrangements, and the rectifier filter from their subsystem list.

The Transducer Design

The overall design of the devices was to be made in such a manner that the acoustic output into the vocal tract be much like or, by using simple electric-drive modifications, shapeable to the laryngeal wave whose place it was taking.

A natural glottal wave has a roughly saw-toothed shape with its associated power spectrum. A good zero-order approximation for transducer-wave generation would be to design one with the capability of making a triangular or saw-toothed sound-pressure wave.

The electrical-driving system imposes some constraints on the transducer design. The simplest and most efficient driver circuit is one that produces periodic short pulses of RF signal, so that after rectification and filtering, a train of short, square-voltage pulses is applied to the transducer. If a transducer with a response to a square wave train that is anything like what is desired can be produced, then proper modification of the driving pulse train can easily modify the acoustic output of the transducer to the desired wave.

So the problem of the production of a proper acoustic signal in the vocal tract becomes that of making a transducer with appropriate mechanical parameters and an acoustic output similar to that desired. Then proper manipulation of the pulsatile, electric-drive signal can synthesize the appropriate vocal-tract wave.

The sort of transducer that we chose to use is the magnetically biased, magnetically actuated type. The cross section of a typical device of this type is shown in Figure 12-1. It consists of an "O"-ring-sealed case with a diaphragm containing a magnetic slug mounted in its center. This slug pulls the very-springy diaphragm downward so that it rests against the pole pieces of the permanent magnet. If the transducer is properly designed, a short pulse of current through the coils produces a subtractive magnetic field,

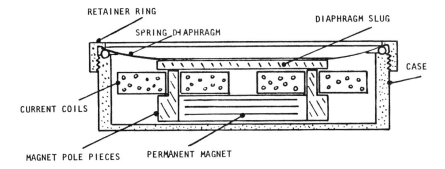

RETAINER RING

DIAPHRAGM SLUG

SPRING DIAPHRAGM

CASE

CURRENT COILS

MAGNET POLE PIECES   PERMANENT MAGNET

Figure 12-1. Cross-section sketch of the implantable electrolaryngeal prosthesis transducer.

nullifying enough of the total magnetic field to allow the slug
and diaphragm to spring completely away from the pole pieces,
go through a ballistic deflection trajectory, and return to rest on
the magnet pole pieces.

The engineering design of such a transducer is complicated.
The force on the magnetic slug from the magnet structure is a
very nonlinear function of spacing between slug and pole piece.
This must be balanced against the nonlinear spring characteristics of the diaphragm in such a way that the slug always returns to
rest on the pole pieces in the absence of coil current.

Following standard design practices, two models of transducers
were produced; the characteristics of the first of these has already
been reported (Bailey 1976). The second of these is what we are
currently using in experiment.

This transducer has a circular cross section, with a post coating
diameter of 1.7 inches and a post coating thickness of 0.375
inches. The maximum excursion of the diaphragm is 0.020 inches,
when excited with an electrical pulse of 7 volts in amplitude with
a pulse width of 2 ms and a pulse-rate frequency of 100/s. The
deflection signal from this device is shown in Figure 12-2, as
measured by the Everett-McConnell technique (McConnell 1974).

To measure the sound-output SPL and wave shape we utilized
the Sondhi tube (Sondhi 1975) in bench measurements on the
transducer unit. These measurements were performed by mounting the transducer at the open end of an SPL-calibrated Sondhi
tube, with a short, airtight coupler. (Use of the Sondhi tube in

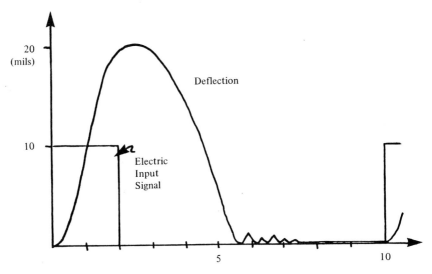

Figure 12-2. Mechanical deflection characteristics of the implantable electro-laryngeal prosthesis transducer.

these measurements will facilitate comparison of pre- and postimplant transducer behavior, because of the projected use of the Sondhi tube in postoperative studies and evaluation).

The sound pressure level (SPL) from this device, as measured into a Sondhi tube, averages over 130 db under the above-cited excitation conditions. This is an inconveniently loud noise, requiring ear mufflers when doing open lab work on the device.

This transducer is fairly efficient in sound generation, and it only requires about three watts of input power for full-sound output.

The tissue-loading capacity of this transducer is also quite acceptable. The release force of the diaphragm upon being pulsed is six pounds. The effect of tissue even up to the maximum estimated weight of 30 gms on the acceleration of the diaphragm is negligible. Thus any attenuation of the acoustic signal (by Sondhi-tube measurement technique), comparing levels before and after transplant, is due to faulty coupling of the vibration from diaphragm to vocal-tract air column.

The Total Implant Unit

Following our initial policy decisions, the implant unit is composed of a electromechanical transducer, power-pickup coil and rectifier-filter section. The power-pickup coil and filter-rectifier section form the power supply for the transducer, which delivers the train of square pulses to the transducer that comes preformed from the extradermal electronic package.

Because of the very poor battery power transfer of the flat inside-coil outside-coil transdermal RF power systems, we soon opted for the toroidal transformer transdermal power-unit configuration. In this configuration, the subdermal coil is wound upon a low-loss, high-magnetic permeability toroidal core. This toroid is then subdermally implanted in such a way that a skin-tunnel passes through the window of the toroid. Connection between the RF transmitter unit and the toroid is made by passing several turns of wire through this skin-lined tunnel through the toroid window and connecting them to the transmitter.

The electromagnetic advantages of this system are highly compensatory. The problem with the flat-coil approach to transdermal RF power transfer is that a large part of the magnetic flux generated by the outside RF transmitter connected coil fails to pass through the subdermal coil. This requires the generation of extremely high magnetic fields in order to transmit power. Since the generation of a high-magnetic field is a very power-wasteful process (outside the cryogenics laboratory), the flat-coil approach is inherently inefficient.

The use of the toroid core is significantly superior. With care in winding the subdermal coil, over 99.7 percent of the magnetic flux generated by the external coil couples into the internal coil. Thus, low losses are incurred in the transmitter, with acceptable overall battery-to-transducer power delivery efficiency.

The subdermal coil is connected to the rectifiers in a way so as to form a simple full-wave rectifier system, with storage capacitor filtering. The pickup toroid and rectifier-filter units are wired together into one functional section, which is connected by a flexible wire to the transducer unit.

Figure 12-3 is a photograph of the present configuration of the

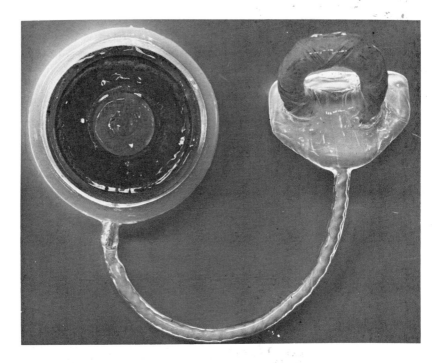

Figure 12-3. The implantable section of the implantable electrolaryngeal prosthesis system. The disc-shaped part is the electromechanical transducer. The rectifier-filter is mounted directly under the transformer toroid.

implant unit. In this figure the unit is back-lighted to show the extent of the encapsulation.

Implant Encapsulation

The implant unit is made of a variety of metals and plastics, so that if it is not protected from the bioambient it will become nonfunctional in a matter of a few days. Conversely, if the bioambient is not protected from the unit, the same thing would happen to it. From the beginning we have relied on encapsulants for isolation.

Silastics in any form proved to be inadequate. Permeability of silastics to ions and water proved to be high enough that unit failure would predictably occur in less than three months, no matter how high the application technology or the beauty of the coating. After passing several years evaluating silastic coating materials and application techniques, the silastics were abandoned, and we had to search for a material with lesser water and ion transport characteristics and less time reactivity.

Finally, we settled on a polyurethane plastic material, Pelethane™, fabricated by the Upjohn Company. It is, with proper procedures, applicable in a layered dip-coating that is uniform, clear and highly protective. Its elastomer qualities are such that transducer encapsulation in coating of 0.030 inch or less does not degrade vibration response. Further, the flexibility of the wires remains adequate.

One of the most vital functions of outer-coating is anchoring. During surgical installation of this unit it is sutured into place, but units that do not have a porous, tissue-impregnable coating as an outside layer readily and rapidly migrate no matter what suturing technique is used. Porous coatings act as beds for tissue ingrowth.

Thickness, pore size, and pore density seem to be the important parameters for the outer coating for this kind of prosthesis.

If the thickness of the porous coating is excessive, the tissue penetration is too great, and fibrous encapsulation is encouraged. For example, many of our early devices were sheathed in Dacron® felt. Within a month the units were encapsulated with over a centimeter of fibrous tissue, and ingrowth was so complete that removal of the unit without severe trauma to the canine subject was impossible.

Coats of about 250μ thickness, with a 10 percent or less total pore area and a pore size of $5\text{-}10\,\mu$, seemed to provide adequate anchorage and has the added benefit that blunt dissection will serve to remove the unit with little or no trauma to the subject. Ideally, one could even remove a malfunctioning unit and slip in a new one in the same surgical procedure without fear of complications.

In our unit the outer coating is provided by a special treatment of the final few dip-coatings, which connect them to a somewhat porous and crater-surfaced porous substance with all of the nice biocompatible characteristics of polyurethane. Ingrowth into this coating limits itself to a tissue coating of several millimeters.

Figure 12-4 is an SEM view of the outside coating of our implant unit.

In the Canadian unit an outer coating of sintered stainless steel provides the anchoring feature. This coating, having more or less the same specifications as ours, provides excellent anchoring and proven easy removability.

Surgical Procedure

The surgical procedure for implantation of the subdermal unit is quite simple in the canine experiments and is easily within the technical ability of any head and neck surgeon. A lateral cervical incision measuring about 8 cm is made, and a combination of sharp and blunt dissection is used to develop a surgical plane, which begins lateral to carotid artery and internal jugular vein and passes deep to these structures and all of the significant neural elements in the midneck. The prevertebral fascia overlying the fifth cervical vertebra is exposed. The transducer unit is

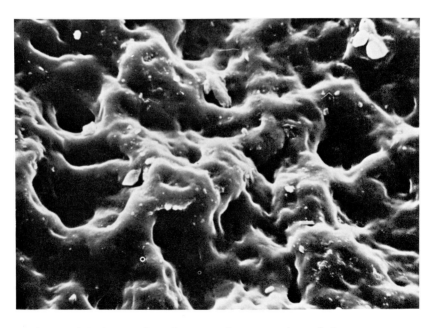

Figure 12-4. A scanning electron microscope view of the outer spongy coating used on the implant section of the electrolaryngeal prosthesis system. The scale here is $1'' = 10 \mu$.

positioned exactly in the midline of this area and sutured to the fascia. A subdermal tunnel is blunt dissected from the retropharyngeal bolsa of the transducer, and the subdermal transformer and its wire is led through it to the power-transfer point. A skin flap is dissected free and used to form a tunnel through the toroid.

The External Electronic Device

The function of the electronic package is to provide the necessary pulsed-power RF signal to the primary (extradermal) winding of the subdermal toroid transformer. The only physical constraint on the device is that it should be small and light. The technical constraint is that it operates at such a frequency that RF losses in the tissue are negligible.

This device has two separate functional aspects. The first is the RF power generator, which transforms battery power to RF carrier power at the required frequency and power level. The second is a set of pulse generators, which provide recurring sets of pulses of variable width and latency. The train of pulse sets are used to key the RF transmitter on and off in such a way as to provide to the transducer with a pulse train that will synthesize the appropriate acoustic output.

The RF section of our device is composed of a class E amplifier. This amplifier uses a tuned circuit as an energy storage system. The energy comes from the battery and is gated into the tuned circuit by a transistor switch. After the tuned circuit is energized, it is allowed to ring, while discharging energy into the load. When the energy in the tuned circuit decreases so that the voltage across the switch is zero, and the current through the tuned circuit inductor is also zero, the switch again gates current into the tuned circuit, and the cycle starts all over again. This form of amplifier is very efficient and converts battery power to RF carrier power with an efficiency easily in excess of 90 percent.

The transistor switch is driven by a simple set of digital timers. One timer generates the appropriate pulse-rate (in pulses per second, pps) and the next tailors this square pulse-train to one with the proper pulse width for keying the switch.

This transmitter is keyed on and off by another set of digital timers. These timers generate periodic pulse sets. The period of the pulse set is at the desired fundamental frequency of the laryngeal signal.

For purposes of canine experiment, we use a simple version of the external electronic package which supplies a periodic, single pulse-train at 100 pps to the transducer. This is because at this time we wish to establish the biocompatibility and reliability of our implant. Along these lines, there is an additional circuit that turns on the systems for 15 seconds, and off for 45 seconds, to mimic human speech patterns, if desired.

This system for the canine experiment is composed of a small electronic package of about 4.5 cubic inches of volume, powered by a large 1.5 ampere-hour rechargable battery. A battery of this capacity will supply power for more than eight hours of continuous uninterrupted speech.

A unit designed for the use of post implant human subjects can be made the size of a pack of cigarettes. This unit, using easily available high-energy density batteries, would have the same or better speech time capabilities as the canine unit.

Acoustic Wave Synthesis

One of the principal thrusts of our research effort is to produce a system within the scope of which is the possibility of speech quality dramatically superior to that of the external prostheses.

To our way of thinking, if we can produce the correct acoustic wave at the proper place in the vocal tract, a human-like speech should result, assuming vocal-tract functionality. Thus, all of the work done and the hardware produced has the capability of ultimately producing an acoustic wave similar, at least in effect, to the human glottal wave (EGW).

The problem of production of an EGW is as follows. Up to this time, and probably into the future, the vibrational sources used will not produce a good EGW with a simple excitation, like, for example, a simple pulse train. What is required is a controlled input that is shaped appropriately, so that the output is the correct shape.

Now the simplest solution to this problem is to provide a varying voltage to the transducer so that the proper response is obtained. This is like the loudspeaker. Application of the proper continuously varying voltage to the loudspeaker causes the loudspeaker to move so as to create the desired sound pressure wave, e.g. music.

This is a solution to the problem of the production of a good EGW, but an expensive one, because production of continuously varying amplitude-modulated RF waves is expensive in terms of power and power efficiency. In order to optimize the ultimate power efficiency of our system and still produce a good EGW, we have opted to use a pulse-train synthesis procedure that is not only compatible with our electronic technique, but cheap to produce even in the ultimate complex form required to produce excellent conformance between the natural glottal wave and the equivalent glottal wave.

The essence of the synthesis of an EGW by pulse trains is shown in Figure 12-5. In Figure 12-5, we see in (*a*) the acoustic output (by means of a Sondhi-tube measurement) due to a simple, periodic square pulse-train excitation of a simple transducer. The wave is very sharp and short and has too high of a high-frequency content. If, as in (*b*), a complex set of periodic square pulses is used, the output of the device is much corrected and the spectrum much more appropriate.

As the number of pulses in the periodic set increase, the approximation of the wave produced to the desired wave can increase so that in the limit, as the number of pulses increase, the error can be made negligible. To determine the correct periodic pulse set that will produce the desired acoustic output from the transducer is the synthesis problem previously mentioned.

Not all physical systems can behave in this way. There are limits on the types of responses that one can expect from a given transducer. However, the transducer that we have produced is designed to produce a wave with a power spectrum, that is a good approximation to that of the natural glottal wave with a reasonable number of pulses in the set.

The amplitude of the wave and its shape are direct functions of the set of periodic pulses that are applied to the transducer. The fundamental pitch is only a function of the periodicity of the pulse sets.

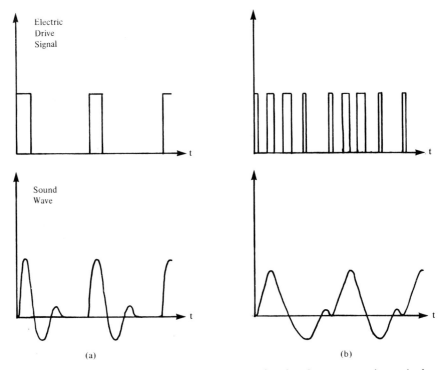

Figure 12-5. (*A*) The sound pressure wave of a simple square train excited electromagnetic transducer; and (*B*) the sound pressure wave of the transducer of part (A), excited by a periodic pulse train to correct waveshape.

Pitch Inflection

Eventually in the humanization of the electrolaryngeal implant speech it will be necessary to effect speech-pitch inflection. This implies a very simple modification of the behavior of the pulse generators in the transmitter control circuitry. However, from whence do we derive the signal which does the deed?

All electrolaryngeal prosthesis devices in common use today derive their control from some sort of manually operated lever or joystick. While this might do as a short-term measure, there are options that we explore in our leisure moments that can be easily implemented to perform the desired operation.

A simple means of deriving a pitch-control signal is to analyze the manner of production of the various vowel sounds. Each vowel sound has a continuum of ways that it can be pronounced and still be recognizable as that particular vowel sound. There have been conducted several series of experiments which show that evaluation of the relative power content of the first formant compared to the power of all of the rest of the formants can provide a useful pitch control signal (Everett, Mitchell, and Yanowitz 1975). Use of this technique implies that the user learns how to modify his vowel pronunciation in such a way as to steer his voice pitch to that desired.

Another useful approach for an implanted electrolaryngeal prosthesis involves a simple frequency analysis of the sound transmitted through lateral or frontal cervical muscles. Voluntary tensing of these muscles provides variable-frequency filtering action of the transmitted sound wave, which may be picked up by a simple contact microphone. Low-band and high-band power content of this signal seems to provide a good signal for pitch-inflection control. It remains to be seen how much the use of these muscles for natural head movements will interfere with their speech function.

A third manner in which pitch control and vibration on-off control may be derived is from the detection of the amplitude of electromyographic (EMG) signals from small, fast, and preferably little-used muscles. The small muscle behind the ears might be utilized. Experience in biofeedback training has shown that muscles such as these are easily placed under very precise control, such that the function becomes almost natural and involuntary.*

Another very satisfactory technique of pitch control and vibration on-off control for an implanted electrolaryngeal prosthesis derives from air pressure or flow from the tracheal stoma of the laryngectomees. (*See* Chapter 7.)

All of these techniques will bear much investigation. However, it would appear that the stoma pressure approach is of such simplicity that its application to the first human recipients of our electrolaryngeal implant is to be expected.

---

*A reviewer from the Canadian group suggested the use of the digastric muscle belly as being the most natural pitch-signal source, assuming that the hyoid bone and its musculature were salvageable.

PROGRESS

To date our group has satisfactorily prototyped all of the hardware for the electrolaryngeal prosthesis system, has developed surgical procedures for the implantation, and has developed acoustic-analysis procedures and acoustic wave synthesis procedures.

Our electronics packages have reached a stage of sophistication such that performance appears to be satisfactory in terms of reliability and performance-output characteristics. Our electronics units are simple to fabricate and easy to align.

A satisfactory configuration for the wireless-excited electrolaryngeal prosthesis implant unit has been produced, and overall satisfactory performance has been obtained from it. Our major stumbling block in the implant unit has been repeated failure from seepage of body fluid into the wires of the unit, because of encapsulant inadequacies. It appears than an adequate encapsulant has been identified, and that the use of Pelethane and the use of glass or ceramic seals on metal enclosures will provide adequate unit lifetime.

Removability of the unit is much simplified by the use of a fine-pored version of Pelethane formed by a special application process.

Surgical-implantation procedures have been standardized and simplified over the past five years. Seroma formation, hematoma formation, and infection are avoided by adherence to standard surgical procedures and routine use of antibiotic therapy. Careful positioning of the transducer in the midline is critical for optimal acoustic coupling from transducer diaphragm to vocal-tract air column. Transducer migration is not a problem during the postoperative period.

We observe in all of our test animals, as does Frederickson (1980), that swallowing is not compromised in spite of obvious projection of the implant transducer into the pharynx. No difficulty in swallowing is expected in human volunteers equipped with an electrolaryngeal prosthesis if the subject has an intact pharyngeal lumen.

Because of the need for examining directly the equivalent glottal wave generated by the electrolaryngeal implant prosthesis, by means of a Sondhi tube, we have taken to measuring the direct output of the electrolaryngeal implant transducer by the same means so as to compare waveshape and total sound pressure output on a before implant - after implant basis.

THE FUTURE

Our current effort is directed at using this, our final year of animal testing, to establish the reliability and durability of the prototype electrolaryngeal prosthesis. Successful completion of these experiments will form the foundation for extension of our project investigations to a small number of carefully selected human volunteers.

REFERENCES

Tait, R.V.: The oral vibrator. *Br Dent J, 106*: 336-340, 1959.

Goode, R.L.: Development of an improved artificial larynx. *Trans Am Acad Ophthalmol Otolaryngol,* 73:279-287, 1969.

Rogers, J.H., Frederickson, J.M., and Bryce, D.P.: New techniques for vocal rehabilitation. *Can J Otolaryngol,* 4:595-604, 1975.

Griffiths, M.V., Frederickson, J.M., and Bryce, D.P.: An implantable electromagnetic sound source for speech production. *Arch Otolaryngol, 102*: 676-682, 1976.

Frederickson, J.M.: Personal Communication, May, 1980.

Bailey, B.J., Everett, R.L., and Griffiths, C.M.: An implanted electronic laryngeal prosthesis. *Am Otol Rhonol Laryngol,* 85(4):472, 1976.

McConnell, J.R.: "A Technique for the Quantitative Recording of Precordial Pulsations." M.S. Thesis, University of Houston, 1974.

Sondhi, M.M.: Measurement of the glottal waveform. *J Acoust Soc Am, 57*: 228-232, 1975.

Everett, R.L., Mitchell, C., and Yanowitz, A.: An Electronic Laryngeal Prosthesis for the Production of Natural Sounding Speech. Proc. 28; *Annual Conf. Eng. in Med. and Biol., 17*:202, 1975.

PART III:
SURGICAL ENHANCEMENT
METHODS

Chapter 13

PARTIAL LARYNGECTOMY PROCEDURES: A REVIEW

BYRON J. BAILEY

ABSTRACT

Vertical partial laryngectomy refers to the group of techniques in which one-half, or more, of the larynx in a vertical dimension is removed. Newer reconstructive techniques permit the rebuilding of the larynx in a manner designed to allow a maximum cancer excision (extended-vertical partial laryngectomy) with preservation of essential sphincteric mechanisms and voice.

Horizontal, or supraglottic, partial laryngectomy is designed to permit the excision of the superior one-half of the larynx. This technique can be extended to include excision of a portion of the base of the tongue or the adjacent pharynx.

It has been established that the control of neoplastic disease is not compromised when proper patient selection is employed, and this issue is discussed. Comments regarding the functional rehabilitation and final outcome of this patient group are reviewed.

INTRODUCTION

A LITTLE OVER a century ago, an imaginative surgeon from New York, Henry B. Sands, performed successfully a laryngotomy for the excision of a glottic carcinoma (Sands 1895). This event heralded the opening of an exciting era of laryngeal surgery, a procedure that continues to change and evolve to the present time.

The objectives that were being pursued by Dr. Sands and that motivated him to embark on this imaginative experiment are very

239

much alive in the minds of today's laryngeal surgeons as they bring sophisticated diagnostic resources to the evaluation of each patient concerning his suitability for "laryngeal-conservation" surgery. The primary goal remains unchanged: the complete removal of all malignant disease. Likewise, the secondary goal continues to be maximum preservation of the respiratory, phonatory, and sphincteric function of the larynx.

The historical developments in the field of laryngeal conservation surgery are fascinating, and one can divide the century between 1870 and 1970 into thirds, each one with a particular distinctive emphasis. The first one-third of that century might be termed a period of "reluctant acceptance of the concept of conservation surgery," and during this period a variety of procedures were devised independently by several pioneers who brought varying degrees of success to their endeavors. In some parts of the world, the concept of conservation surgery was buried and resurrected on several occasions.

The second-third of this period of time would coincide with the first forty years of the twentieth century. During this particular period there was a great deal of information disseminated throughout the medical literature: it was a period of popularization and basic development. During this time, the pioneer laryngeal-conservation surgeons provided convincing evidence of the soundness of their observations and conclusions that this was a safe and useful concept. Much was learned concerning the proper selection of cases, and a few standardized extirpative procedures such as *hemilaryngectomy* and *laryngofissure* were reported and gained popularity.

The last part of this period (the past 40 years) has been of refinement and widespread acceptance of these techniques. The more general medical advances, such as antibiotic therapy, improved general anesthesia, and better techniques for blood replacement have permitted us to enjoy an era of modern surgery and increased surgical safety. We have learned a great deal more, with regard to the clarification of the indications for and the limitations of conservation surgery, and there has been a recent important emphasis on reconstructive procedures (laryngoplasty procedures) that are designed to enhance the preservation of function.

It is the purpose of this presentation to focus on the issue of *vertical partial laryngectomy* and to trace its origins, its basic science foundations, and its emerging role in the field of laryngeal cancer surgery. The issues and techniques that we will address will move away from the central theme of this particular meeting and must be viewed in the context that "function preserved is function that does not require restoration." It is hoped that this information will broaden the perspective of readers much as so many of the other chapters have broadened the perspective of this author.

HISTORICAL REVIEW

The evolution of the concept and specific procedures of partial laryngectomy are traced in Table 13-I from their origins in the nineteenth century (Bailey 1971). We can see that the process began with experiments in the animal laboratory of H. Albers in 1829 and moved from there to surgical investigations and observations. These exercises preceded a clear understanding of the pathophysiology of laryngeal cancer and even of the anatomical basis for conservation surgery, which lies in the unique configuration of the lymphatic circulatory system of the human larynx.

This evolutionary process was rooted in the fertile soil of keen minds and careful clinical observation. It is a historical chapter in the development of surgery that is not without its darker moments, such as the serious international political controversies that surrounded the management of the laryngeal cancer of Prince Frederick. It is also important to remember that this evolution in its early years was occurring at a time when even the concept of medical specialization was under serious attack, and those who indicated to their colleagues that they specialized only in diseases of the larynx were viewed by many skeptics as being only one-step above the status of a medical charlatan.

In spite of the obstacles that we might have difficulty in surmounting today, progress was made, and each successive decade built upon the strengths and worked to overcome the weaknesses of the prior decade.

Over time, a clear picture has emerged that documents both the

Table 13-I. Events in the Evolution, Popularization, and Investigation of
Conservation Cancer Surgery of the Larynx

100 A. D.	Araeteus was the first to write about cancer of the larynx.
1732	Morgagni described the autopsies of two deaths from cancer of the larynx.
1788	Pelletan performed the first external surgical approach to larynx. This was done for the removal of a foreign body.
1810	Desault described the operation, "laryngotomy."
1829	H. Albers performed experimental partial and total laryngectomies in dogs.
1863	H. B. Sands performed the first partial laryngectomy for cancer. The patient was a 30-year-old female who survived 2 years and died of cancer of the kidney without laryngeal recurrence.
1864	Duncan Gibbs removed an epidermoid carcinoma via laryngotomy in a 29-year-old female patient. She developed a recurrence one year postoperatively.
1865	Sir Astley Cooper removed a malignant tumor of the epiglottis by finger dissection by a transoral approach.
1866	Patrick Heron Watson. He performed the first total laryngectomy. This was done for a patient with laryngeal syphilis.
1870	V. Czerny. His interest in Watson's laryngectomy led him to perform surgical experiments in dogs. He assisted Billroth on the first laryngectomy performed for cancer.
1873	T. Billroth. Billroth was the first to perform total laryngectomy for cancer. The patient was a thirty-six-year-old male who developed local recurrence and died seven months postoperatively.
1875	T. Billroth. He reported a case in which he performed a hemilaryngectomy for cancer.
1876	E. Isambert. Isambert reported his results in five cases of cancer of the larynx treated by partial laryngectomy. He also classified laryngeal tumors using the terms "intrinsic," "extrinsic," and "subglottic."
1891	J. Hajek. Hajek reported studies of laryngeal lymphatics which would support the concept of partial laryngectomy.
1903	Felix Semon. In a series of eighteen cases of thyrotomy, Semon reported that fifteen of these patients were cured at one or more years.
1904	P. R. W. de Sancti. He reported studies of laryngeal lymphatics and their importance in regard to cancer.
1909	Henry Butlin. In a series of twenty-one patients who had laryngofissure, Butlin reported that there was only one operative death, and seventeen patients were alive and well three years postoperatively.
1912	St. Clair Thompson. This was reported as a series of ten laryngofissures. There was no operative mortality; one patient died of recurrence and one later required a total laryngectomy. There were eight patients reported cured.
1912	Gluck and Sörenson. They described a standard technique for hemilaryngectomy.
1916	L. H. Lack. Described here was a technique extending cordectomy to include a portion of the overlying thyroid cartilage.
1922-1930	St. Clair Thompson. Thompson wrote a series of articles that simplified and standardized the laryngofissure procedure. He reported 70 cases with a 76 percent, three-year cure rate.
1930	A. Hautant. He published his experience with a modification of the hemilaryngectomy of Gluck and Sörenson and reported twenty cases with two operative deaths.

Table 13-I continued.

1940	L. H. Clerf. He described modified partial laryngectomy for anterior commissure carcinoma.
1943	E. N. Broyles. Described here were the histologic features of the anterior commissure tendon and its clinical significance in anterior commissure carcinoma.
1947	J. M. Alonso. He described partial vertical laryngectomy for selected lesions involving the pyriform sinus and partial horizontal laryngectomy for supraglottic malignancy.
1951	M. L. Som. Som described the use of sliding mucosal flaps to close the defect after hemilaryngectomy.
1954	J. J. Pressman. Pressman reported a technique for partial laryngectomy wherein one or both thyroid alae are removed and then replaced in a muscular pocket to restore laryngeal support, and the lumen of the larynx is lined with perichondrium. He also reported basic observations regarding the "compartmentation" of the laryngeal lymphatics.
1956	J. Leroux Robert. He described the "extended fronto-lateral" partial laryngectomy, which allows resection of more extensive malignant lesions.
1956	M. L. Som. Som described a technique for partial laryngoesophagectomy.
1958	J. H. Ogura. He modified a horizontal partial laryngectomy, which eliminated the need for a pharyngostoma.
1960	J. H. Ogura. Ogura refined the technique for partial laryngopharyngectomy with radical neck dissection for pyriform sinus lesions.
1962	J. Miodonski. His results with an extended hemilaryngectomy, which includes partial removal of the cricoid cartilage and the epiglottis, were reported.
1965	J. H. Ogura. Ogura reported a technique utilizing a cartilaginous triangle from the superior rim of the thyroid cartilage to reconstruct the glottis after partial laryngectomy.
1967	Bernstein and Holt. They described the use of the bipedicle sternohyoid muscle flap as a "filler" in cases of uncompensated unilateral vocal cord paralysis.
1968	Maran et al. This group reported experimental results in a variety of laryngoplasty techniques, which included bipedicle sternohyoid muscle laryngoplasty.
1969	H. Quinn. Quinn described the use of free-muscle grafts for glottic reconstruction after partial laryngectomy.
1969	J. E. Delahunty et al. Reported here were the results of vocal cord transplantation in dogs.
1969	J. H. Ogura and H. Biller. These two reported on the use of a monopedicle sternohyoid muscle flap for glottic reconstruction after partial laryngectomy.

safety and efficacy of vertical partial laryngectomy, extended-vertical laryngectomy, and supraglottic partial laryngectomy. The concept of laryngoplasty to augment the surgical defect created by the extirpative portion of the operation is also gaining more widespread acceptance as a technique designed to maximize the conservation of function.

TECHNIQUE OF VERTICAL PARTIAL
LARYNGECTOMY AND LARYNGOPLASTY

It has been shown that the majority of malignant tumors in the larynx arise on the margin of the true vocal cord and spread from this site by direct extension and through lymphatic pathways. The concept of compartments of laryngeal lymphatics was pursued by Hajek (1891). More recently, these findings have been confirmed and expanded by the work of Pressman (1956), who employed sophisticated techniques of dye and radioisotopic tracers. These studies have shown that the laryngeal lymphatics can be divided into four quadrants, separated by the laryngeal midline vertically and by the superior margin of the true vocal cord horizontally. Carcinoma arising on one vocal cord tends to remain localized to that quadrant and does not spread superiorly nor across the midline of the larynx. Malignancy arising above the level of the true vocal cords tends to metastasize in a superior and lateral direction rather than to spread inferiorly.

Thus, we can see that for glottic carcinoma (the most common type), a procedure that preserves one-half of the larynx is theoretically a safe procedure in terms of cancer surgery. An operative technique that removes the top half of the larynx as part of the management for a supraglottic lesion should provide the safety required in terms of adequate clearance of the margin of the tumor.

The technique that we present here is a modification that incorporates the principles of laryngeal reconstruction that were originally developed by Pressman (1954). It was his observation that many tumors of the larynx can be removed without sacrificing the thyroid cartilage, and that the preservation of this cartilage is of value in the reconstructive phase of the surgical procedure. While Pressman originally excised the thyroid alae completely from the operative field and then replaced them into muscular pockets that were created surgically after the tumor removal, the author's modification preserves the intact attachment of the thyroid alae posteriorly and employs a bipedicle muscle flap for the reconstructive phase.

The technique will be illustrated in two forms: the first is a simple unilateral technique for lesions that do not encroach upon the anterior commissure (the location within the larynx where the two true vocal cords meet anteriorly); and, the second is a modification of this, which is suitable for the management of lesions that involve both true vocal cords and the anterior commissure.

PRELIMINARY TRACHEOTOMY. Local anesthesia is used to accomplish a tracheotomy through an incision that is approximately 8 centimeters in length and is located about 2 centimeters inferior to the margin of the cricoid cartilage. An endotracheal tube is inserted and general inhalation anesthesia is then induced.

SKIN INCISION. The original tracheotomy incision is then extended laterally following major skin creases in the neck as shown in Figure 13-1. An anterior neck flap consisting of skin and platysma muscle is elevated to a point just above the hyoid bone and is retracted superiorly and protected with moist saline dressings.

EXPLORATION OF THE LYMPHATIC NODE SYSTEM. The surgical dissection is carried deep to the sternocleidomastoid muscles on each side in the inferior and midportion of the neck, and the carotid sheath is exposed. This permits the surgeon to palpate the cervical chain of nodes and to inspect them for the possibility of malignancy as shown in Figure 13-2. Early metastatic deposits might otherwise be overlooked, and they are, in the opinion of this author, a contraindication to vertical partial laryngectomy. While there are some who would perform a vertical partial laryngectomy in the presence of a cervical lymph node metastasis, it is felt by many that this would be an unacceptable compromise in terms of the primary objective (the adequate management of the carcinoma), because this is an objective that takes precedence over the secondary issues of preservation of function.

ELEVATION OF EXTERNAL PERICHONDRIUM OF THE THYROID CARTILAGE. A vertical midline incision is made and a plane is developed between the two sternohyoid muscles and through the external perichondrial layer of the thyroid cartilage. This is connected superiorly to curved incisions that are made along the superior margin of the alae of the thryoid cartilage. Paired

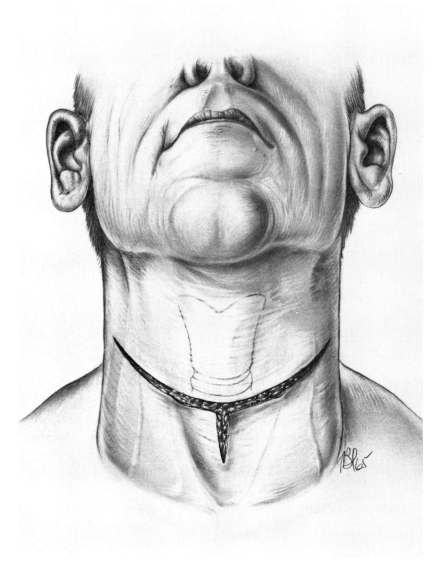

Figure 13-1. A curved, transverse cervical incision at the level of the second tracheal ring is made in order to accomplish the tracheotomy and obtain the necessary exposure. Reprinted with permission from the *Transactions of the American Academy of Opthalmology and Otolaryngology*, July-August:561, 1966.

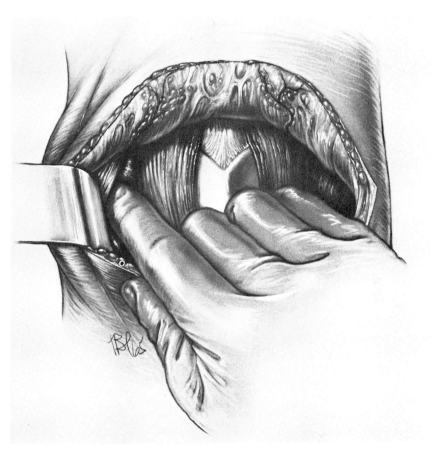

Figure 13-2. The anterior neck is palpated for possible metastatic carcinoma in cervical lymph nodes. Reprinted with permission from the *Transactions of the American Academy of Ophthalmology and Otolaryngology*, July-August:561, 1966.

incisions are also made along the inferior margin of the perichondrium and are carried out laterally to the region of the inferior cornua. The external perichondrium is then elevated very carefully back to the origin of the superior and inferior cornua of the thyroid cartilage on the side of tumor involvement. Great care is taken by the surgeon to avoid tearing or inadvertently lacerating the external perichondrial layer, as this tissue is vital to the lining of the larynx following the surgical resection and reconstruction. The medial margin of the perichondrium is fixed to the deep surface of the medial margin of the sternohyoid muscle as shown in Figure 13-3. This is a maneuver that greatly

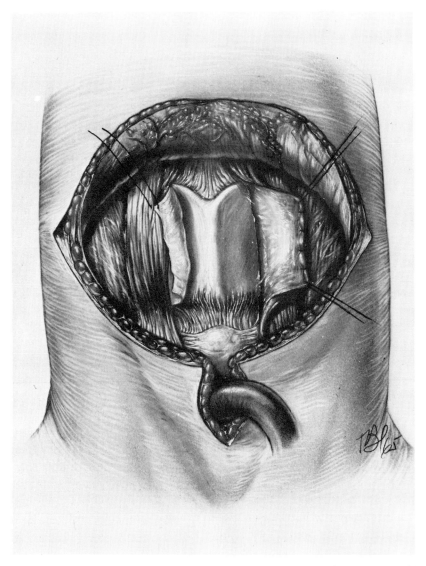

Figure 13-3. The external perichondrium is elevated away from the thyroid cartilage. Reprinted with permission from the *Transactions of the American Academy of Ophthalmology and Otolaryngology*, July-August:562, 1966.

facilitates the elevation and preservation of the perichondrium and also eliminates the necessity of working with loose tissue that could be torn or that could diminish in size by shrinkage.

THYROTOMY. The investigations conducted by Broyles (1943) have shown that the vocalis muscle tendon attaches directly into the substance of the thyroid cartilage in the region of the anterior commissure and that there is no perichondrial layer at this point. It is impossible, therefore, to perform a true subperichondrial dissection in this area. This unusual anatomical arrangement is responsible, in part, for a higher incidence of persistent and recurrent carcinoma when the primary lesion extends to involve the anterior commissure of the larynx. It also forms the anatomical basis for the bilateral thyrotomy procedures of Kemler (1947), Clerf (1940) and Leroux-Robert (1956). When the lesion does not encroach upon the anterior commissure region, the larynx can be entered safely in the midline. Incisions are then made horizontally across the midportion of the false vocal cord and along the inferior margin of the thyroid cartilage, and the larynx can then be opened and inspected. Tumor resection is accomplished by meticulous elevation of the internal perichondrium of the thyroid cartilage. The steps in the resection are shown in Figures 13-4, 13-5, 13-6, and 13-7.

Thin strips of the epithelial margins are then taken from the edges of the excision and sent to the pathologist for frozen-section examination in order to be certain that the carcinoma has been adequately excised.

LARYNGOPLASTY. The second portion of the operative procedure is focused upon reconstruction as a surgical step in vocal rehabilitation. A bipedicle muscle flap is isolated and repositioned inside the thyroid ala in order to replace the tissue that has been removed in the extirpative phase of the operation (*see* Figure 13-8, 13-9, and 13-10). The laryngeal lumen is thereby lined with the tissue layer that was formerly elevated from the outer surface of the thyroid cartilage (external perichondrial layer). The perichondrial margins are sutured to the remaining mucosal margins inside the larynx as part of the closure, and then the larynx itself is closed by approximating the two thyroid alae to each other, using stabilizing suture of 2-0 chromic catgut (*see* Figure 13-11).

Healing and recovery may be enhanced by the use of a laryngeal

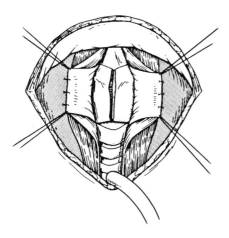

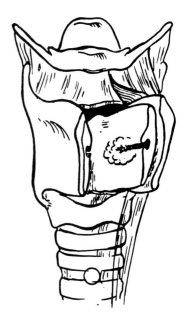

Figure 13-4. The thyroid cartilage is divided in the midline, with care being taken to avoid entering the laryngeal lumen.

Figure 13-5. After elevating the internal perichondrium of the thyroid cartilage, the larynx is entered and the tumor is visualized. Reprinted with permission from the *Laryngoscope, 81*(11):1742-1771, 1971.

stent or an anterior commissure keel. Management of granulation tissue must be accomplished in order to prevent scarring, web formation, and postoperative laryngeal stenosis.

BILATERAL RESECTION AND RECONSTRUCTION. The unique anatomical features of the anterior commissure have been reviewed, and their clinical significance is sufficient to warrant a modification when carcinoma is present at or near the anterior commissure of the larynx. The midline thyrotomy incision that is appropriate for a unilateral tumor would risk surgical violation of the carcinoma during the entry to the laryngeal lumen that is required for tumor visualization. As shown in Figure 13-12, bilateral, paramedian incisions are made approximately five millimeters from the midline, thereby creating a central strip of thyroid cartilage. Through these bilateral incisions, the internal perichondrium can be elevated from the thyroid alae, and the laryngeal lumen is entered well away from the margin of the malignancy.

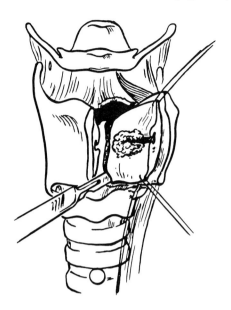

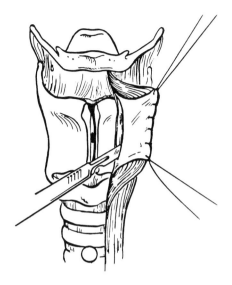

Figure 13-6. The tumor is resected along with an adequate margin of normal tissue. The specimen includes the entire true vocal cord and most of the false vocal cord. Reprinted with permission from the *Laryngoscope, 81*(11): 1742-1771, 1971.

Figure 13-7. An incision is made to create a bipedicle sternohyoid muscle flap with perichondrium on its deep surface. Reprinted with permission from the *Laryngoscope, 81*(11):1742-1771, 1971.

The larynx is entered on the side of less involvement (*see* Figure 13-13) with the tumor, and it is imperative that the arytenoid cartilage be spared on that particular side if an adequately functioning larynx is to be preserved. It is possible from this point of entry to work around the circumference of the neoplasm and to open the larynx gradually and gain full visual and surgical control of the tumor. The resection is then accomplished en bloc with the soft tissue still attached to the midline cartilage strip (*see* Figure 13-14).

Once again, frozen-section margins are obtained to confirm the adequacy of the surgical procedure.

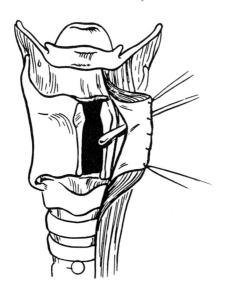

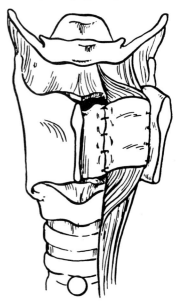

Figure 13-8. The muscle flap is repositioned to the interior of the larynx (deep to the thyroid cartilage). Reprinted with permission from the *Laryngoscope, 81*(11):1742-1771, 1971.

Figure 13-9. The muscle flap is repositioned within the larynx and the mucosa is sutured to the perichondrium. Reprinted with permission from the *Laryngoscope, 81*(11):1742-1771, 1971.

This technique permits an excision that can include as much as three-quarters of the circumference of the larynx in order to include virtually all of the true vocal cord and false vocal cord area (on the side of greater tumor involvement) and two-thirds of the contralateral true and false cords. One arytenoid cartilage and the posterior commissure of the larynx must be preserved if adequate postoperative function is to be maintained.

Bilateral, bipedicle muscle flaps with the attached external thyroid perichondrium are then developed and repositioned to the interior of the thyroid alae (*see* Figure 13-15). A soft-plastic or rubber stent is recommended routinely in the case of bilateral laryngoplasty procedures.

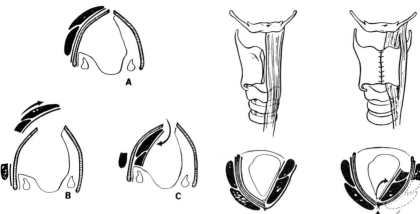

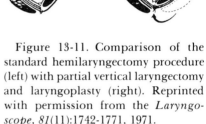

Figure 13-10. Diagram of the repositioned bipedicle flap in order to accomplish the laryngoplasty reconstruction. Reprinted with permission from the *Laryngoscope, 81*(11):1742-1771, 1971.

Figure 13-11. Comparison of the standard hemilaryngectomy procedure (left) with partial vertical laryngectomy and laryngoplasty (right). Reprinted with permission from the *Laryngoscope, 81*(11):1742-1771, 1971.

SUPRAGLOTTIC PARTIAL LARYNGECTOMY

Epidermoid carcinoma of the larynx, the most frequently encountered laryngeal malignancy, may be located entirely above the level of the true vocal cords. In the event of limited extension outside the confines of the larynx, a patient with this geographic location of the primary may be a favorable candidate for supraglottic partial laryngectomy.

The lymphatic circulation in the supraglottic region differs from that at the level of the glottis in that there is a much greater tendency for tumor spread to cross the midline. These primary tumors also have a tendency to metastasize to ipsilateral and

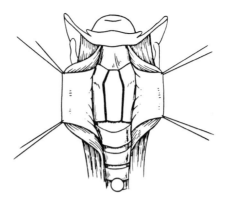

Figure 13-12. Bilateral paramedian incisions of the thyroid cartilage create a "central segment" in the presence of tumor involving the anterior commissure.

contralateral lymph nodes more frequently and earlier in the course of the disease. Because the patient with supraglottic carcinoma will usually *not* present with hoarseness early in the course of disease, some of our impressions concerning supraglottic carcinoma may tend to underestimate the length of time that cancer has been present.

Another feature unique to the conservation surgery of supraglottic carcinoma is that it is entirely practical to combine supraglottic partial laryngectomy with surgical excision of cervical lymph nodes that are invaded by metastatic carcinoma cells. Traditionally, this involved performance of a standard radical neck dissection, but in more recent years, the conservation of major neck structures has gained acceptance.

EXPOSURE OF THE LARYNX. Tracheotomy is usually the first step in this technique and may be performed under local or general anesthesia. The larynx is exposed by raising an apron flap of anterior cervical skin and platysma muscle, or by intersecting midline horizontal and lateral vertical incisions, which resemble a "T" lying on its side. The midline strap muscles are visualized and are divided near the hyoid bone and reflected anteriorly and inferiorly. An incision is then made in the

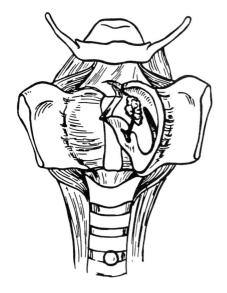 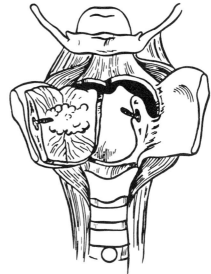

Figure 13-13. The larynx is entered on the side of lesser tumor involvement. Reprinted with permission from the *Laryngoscope*, *81*(11):1742-1771, 1971.

Figure 13-14. As the dissection is continued, complete visualization of the tumor is accomplished and a resection of one entire half of the larynx and one half of the opposite side of the larynx is accomplished.

perichondrium along the superior border of the thyroid cartilage.

PERICHONDRIAL ELEVATION. The external perichondrium of the thyroid cartilage is then elevated very carefully from the superior two-thirds of the thyroid cartilage. Just as in the case of vertical partial laryngectomy, the perichondrium is an extremely important layer in the postresection closure phase of the operative procedure. A blunt elevator and cotton "peanut" dissector permit the careful elevation of this layer without laceration of the perichondrium.

CARTILAGE INCISION. The thyroid cartilage is transected approximately halfway between the inferior extent of the superior midline notch of the thyroid cartilage and the inferior margin of the thyroid cartilage in the midline. Care is taken to

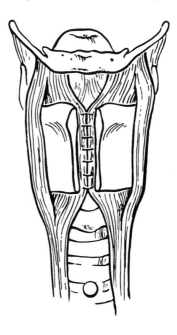

Figure 13-15. Reconstruction
of the larynx using bilateral, bipedicle muscle flaps. Reprinted
with permission from the *Laryngoscope, 81*(11):1742-1771, 1971.

avoid extensive laceration and tearing of the intralaryngeal soft
tissue when the motorized saw is used to make this cut. It is the
intent of the surgeon to transect the larynx just above the superior
margin of the true vocal cords.

HYOID BONE DISSECTION. The suprahyoid musculature is
then transected from its attachment to the hyoid bone, and the
dissection in this area is carried down to permit entry into the
lateral portion of the hypopharynx at the level of the epiglottis.
The exposure is increased by dissecting across the vallecula just
above the level of the hyoid until the supraglottic region can be
visualized easily.

TUMOR RESECTION. The epiglottis is grasped in an instrument
and retracted superiorly and forward. This permits a resection

that continues from the lateral pharyngeal wall across to the larynx on each side and then passes just superior to the arytenoid cartilages and downward toward the attachment of the epiglottis, immediately above the anterior commissure area. The intralaryngeal transection lines are then connected to the external cartilage cuts at the level of the laryngeal ventricles, and the specimen is then removed en bloc and in continuity with unilateral or bilateral neck dissection specimens, if any have been necessary.

CRICOPHARYNGEAL MYOTOMY. Although there has been some controversy regarding the importance or necessity for cricopharyngeal myotomy, it still is a popular adjunctive step in this surgical procedure. Cricopharyngeal myotomy is accomplished by inserting the finger into the hypopharynx and dissecting slowly down through the inferior constrictor muscle until the gloved finger can be seen through the remaining hypopharyngeal-superior esophageal mucosa. The rationale behind this step is that the ability to swallow without aspirating will be enhanced postoperatively.

CLOSURE. The surgeon then confirms by frozen-section margins that the tumor has been adequately resected and that the vocal cord motion is still intact. Closure is accomplished by one row of heavy sutures that are placed between the external thyroid perichondrial flap and the muscle at the base of the tongue. Closure is accomplished in three or four layers in an effort to obtain a completely watertight seal. The postoperative rehabilitation of the patient with supraglottic laryngectomy is ordinarily uneventful in terms of vocal function. The time and effort required to rehabilitate the function of swallowing in association with the sphincteric protective function of the larynx varies quite widely. The regimen ordinarily begins with soft foods and/or carbonated beverages, as these are somewhat easier to swallow for most patients. When the temperature of the liquid is quite cool or warm it is easier for the patient to feel the foreign material and avoid aspiration. Within a period of time that usually ranges from three weeks to three months, most patients will have regained the ability to swallow without significant aspiration, and very few will experience more than a minor functional inconvenience by six months.

OBSERVATIONS

As mentioned previously, the last thirty years have been a period of general acceptance for surgical-conservation procedures involving the larynx. The initial tendency for some enthusiastic surgeons to push these procedures beyond their reasonable limits and the reluctance of other surgeons to accept them under any circumstances has gradually faded. There is considerable agreement concerning the indications for employing conservation procedures and general acceptance of the fact that when appropriate patient selection is employed, the cancer control capability of these procedures equals that of total laryngectomy and exceeds that of radiation therapy.

We have recently analyzed our series of seventy patients with laryngeal carcinoma who have undergone vertical partial laryngectomy between the years of 1960 through 1978. Ten of these patients were operated upon less than two years ago and are excluded from some of our comments that will follow, in view of the fact that time has been too short to permit statistical evaluation. In some instances, the entire group will be discussed when followup is not an issue.

As mentioned previously, none of the patients in our series had cervical lymph node metastasis at the time of surgery. The primary laryngeal lesion involved the mobile portion of the true vocal cord (4 patients), the arytenoid cartilage vocal process (10 patients), the anterior commissure (45 patients), and transglottic lesions (involving the false cord ventricle and true vocal cord) were present in eleven patients.

Analysis of treatment outcome shows that of the sixty patients who are more than two years postoperative from vertical partial laryngectomy, four (6.7%) are dead of causes other than cancer during the first five years of followup. Five patients (8.3%) are deceased from causes related to cancer, but three of these patients developed a second primary carcinoma involving the lung, and only two are dead of causes related to their original carcinoma. Eight patients (13.3%) in the group were found to have recurrent laryngeal carcinoma, but six of these have been salvaged and are alive and well with no evidence of carcinoma. Salvage was accomplished by a second, partial-laryngectomy procedure in one instance, by radiation therapy in two instances, and by total laryngectomy in three instances.

Complications following vertical partial laryngectomy have been relatively infrequent. Laryngeal stenosis (narrowing of the airway) occurred in four patients, but was mild in two of these (symptomatic only on marked physical exertion). Of the two patients with moderate to severe stenosis, one required tracheotomy but otherwise functions normally without exercise restriction, and the other appears to have a psychological dependence upon her tracheotomy.

Only one patient in the series developed a serious postoperative infection and that person had a prolonged period of laryngeal edema, but was decannulated at about three months postoperatively.

Aspiration of saliva and food has been a minor problem in many patients during the first few days after the reinstitution of per oral alimentation. This phenomenon is often related to the wearing of a tracheotomy tube with its associated disturbance in the normal intrathoracic pressure differential associated with swallowing. Aspiration has persisted beyond a few days in only two patients, lasting approximately three weeks in one patient, and six weeks in another, but has not resulted in a postoperative pneumonia in any of the patients. Abnormality of vocal quality has been present in all patients in this series. Their hoarseness has been characterized by excessive breathiness, a moderately harsh vocal quality, diminished pitch range, diminished phonation time, and decreased volume. It is the opinion of the author that vocal quality with this procedure is superior to the vocal quality associated with standard hemilaryngectomy (without laryngoplasty), but is not as satisfactory as postradiation voice therapy. There have been no instances, however, in which the vocal quality has been compromised to the extent that it has interfered with the patient's social, psychological, or economic well-being. The patients in this series, while commenting occasionally upon their vocal change, have indicated their satisfaction and have not felt that their altered vocal quality should be characterized as "a problem." Patients are counseled extensively preoperatively and postoperatively by both surgeon and speech pathologist, and this may be a factor in the observations we are reporting. The author feels strongly that the speech pathologist/therapist has a great deal to offer in terms of assisting the patient in the obtaining of maximum vocal output postoperatively.

Overall, the analysis of our results has been extremely satisfactory in terms of cancer management. Of the sixty patients who are more than two years postoperative, there has been control of the primary carcinoma in fifty-two (86.7%). Fifty-five patients in this series have survived their cancer for more than five years (or have died from noncancer causes), for a cancer survival rate of 91.7 percent.

Looking broadly at the entire group of seventy patients, there are fifty-three who are alive and well with no evidence of carcinoma and who are living with laryngeal function basically intact following partial laryngectomy, plus an additional three patients alive and well with no evidence of carcinoma following total laryngectomy salvage. Of the entire group of seventy patients, there are only twenty-four who are no longer under active followup. Four patients were lost to followup at five to ten years postoperatively, and twenty patients were lost to followup after a minimum of ten years followup.

These results are comparable to the statistics reported by other observers. For example, in 1974 Sessions (1976) reported that one of every four patients with laryngeal carcinoma involving the glottis was found to have secondary extension of the tumor to the anterior commissure region. In the series of sixty-one patients with carcinoma involving the true vocal cord in which there was extension to the anterior commissure, the surgical treatment with hemilaryngectomy resulted in an absolute survival rate of 74 percent. Som and Silver (1968) reported a series of thirty-eight patients with similar glottic carcinoma in which they achieved a three-year survival rate of 68 percent employing hemilaryngectomy. Various studies in which radiation therapy has been employed for comparable anterior commissure lesions report cure rates that vary from 46-74 percent.

Therefore, it seems reasonable to conclude that surgical treatment with vertical partial laryngectomy appears to offer some advantage over radiation therapy in terms of curability. The addition of laryngoplasty following partial laryngectomy seems to provide enhanced preservation of laryngeal function as it relates to phonation, respiration, and swallowing.

The same general pattern of excellent cancer control and preservation of laryngeal function applies to the observations noted following supraglottic partial laryngectomy for carcinoma. The lymphatic system crossover and the rich network of superior cervical lymphatics necessitates the removal of the entire supraglottic portion of the larynx and the more frequent use of cervical node dissection. In spite of the more extensive surgery employed, recovery from supraglottic partial laryngectomy is usually fairly rapid and uneventful if the patient has not received previous radiation therapy. The process of compensation for the loss of the protective function of the superior one-half of the larynx should be assisted by an active rehabilitation program. Phonatory function is excellent in most cases, with the exception of some lowering of vocal pitch and reduction in pitch range.

Once again, careful patient selection for this procedure is the key to a successful outcome in the majority of patients. Long-term cure rates have been equivalent to those achieved by total laryngectomy and are superior to the results achieved from radiation therapy when used alone. This degree of efficacy, coupled with the safety and preservation of function, have assured supraglottic partial laryngectomy of a very important role in the management of laryngeal cancer.

SUMMARY

The above information has been compiled as general background material for the nonsurgical speech scientist in an effort to provide a broader perspective for those working in this expanding interdisciplinary area. It seems likely that the 1980s will be an exciting decade in terms of anticipated advances and improvements that will be provided on many fronts for patients who have become the victims of laryngeal cancer.

REFERENCES

Bailey, B.J.: Partial Laryngectomy and laryngoplasty. *Laryngoscope, 81* (11): 1742-1771, 1971.

Broyles, E.N.: The anterior commissure tendon. *Ann Otol Rhinol Laryngol,* 52:342-345, 1943.

Clerf, L.H.: Cancer of the larynx: an analysis of 250 operative cases. *Arch Otolaryngol, 32*:484-498, 1940.

Hajek, J.: Anatomische untersuchungen uber das larynxodem. *Arch Klin Chir, 42*: 46-93, 1891.

Kemler, J.I.: Bilateral thyrotomy for carcinoma of the larynx. *Laryngoscope,* 57:704-718, 1947.

Leroux-Robert, J.: Indications for radical surgery, partial surgery, radiotherapy, and combined surgery and radiotherapy for cancer of the larynx and hypopharynx. *Ann Otol, 65*:137-153, 1956.

Pressman, J.J.: Cancer of the larynx: laryngoplasty to avoid laryngectomy. *Arch Otolaryngol, 59*:395-412, 1954.

_____: Submucosal compartmentation of the larynx. *Ann Otol Rhinol Laryngol, 65*:766-971, 1956.

Sands, H.B.: Case of cancer of the larynx, successfully removed by laryngotomy; with an analysis of 50 cases of tumors of the larynx, treated by operation. *NY Med J, 1*: 110-126, 1895.

Sessions, D.B., Ogura, J.H., and Fried, M.G.: Laryngeal Carcinoma Involving Anterior Commissure and Subglottis. *Workshops from the Centennial Conference on Laryngeal Cancer.* Alberti, P.M., and Bryce, D.P. (Eds.). New York: Appleton-Century-Crofts, 1976, pp. 674-678.

Som, M.L., and Silver, D.C.: The anterior commissure technique of partial laryngectomy. *Arch Otolaryngol, 87*:138-145, 1968.

RECONSTRUCTIVE SUBTOTAL LARYNGECTOMY WITH VOICE PRESERVATION FOR T3 LARYNGEAL CARCINOMA

BRUCE W. PEARSON, DAVID E. HARTMAN, ROBERT D. WOODS

ABSTRACT

For unilateral invasive squamous cell carcinomas that fix one side of the larynx but spare the pharynx, total laryngectomy has often been employed. In many instances, however, the loss of voice that follows total laryngectomy is unnecessary, as the uninvolved portions of the larynx can be readily used in the construction of a tracheopharyngeal fistula for voice production.

Ten *consecutive* cases, nine T3 laryngeal carcinomas (four glottic, two transglottic, one supraglottic, one subglottic, and one pyriform) and one sarcoma, treated by a new reconstructive subtotal laryngectomy technique have achieved satisfactory voice. Follow-up examination of all patients has revealed (1) average subglottic pressures of 25 ±6 cm of water (threshold opening) and 43 ±20 cm of water (for phonation), and (2) no significant aspiration.

The reconstructive principle involves creation of a tracheopharyngeal fistula, which functions as a neoglottis for phonation, but constricts during swallowing. On the uninvolved side of the larynx, the recurrent and superior laryngeal nerves, and the myomucosal segment of intrinsic laryngeal musculature to which they are attached, are preserved in continuity with the trachea and the pyriform fossa. By releasing these soft tissues from their associated cartilaginous support, the myomucosal segment acquires the flaccidity necessary to form a mucosal-lined tube. The diameter of the tube is increased by supplementing the construction with a flap of hypopharyngeal mucosa from the opposite side.

The technique offers several advantages over existing vocal-reconstruction procedures. It is easily done at the time of primary excision and only involves a single-stage operation. Also, it provides excellent intraoperative visualization

263

of the tumor, and if deemed necessary, it allows conversion to wider-field laryngectomy, partial laryngopharyngectomy, or conventional hemilaryngectomy. It does not compromise the patient's option to learn esophageal voice. The mucosal-lined shunt is self-cleaning and is innervated by the remaining recurrent and superior laryngeal nerves, thus providing a mechanism for constriction during swallowing. With the exception of a tracheostomy tube, no external apparatus is required for respiration or phonation.

The disadvantages of the technique include an additional thirty minutes of surgery and the necessity for the patient to use a hand to valve the tracheal stoma to talk. Because of difficulty in judging radiocurrent tumor margins with accuracy, the technique is probably not suitable for patients who have undergone extensive radiation treatment. It can be employed only at the time of primary laryngectomy and is therefore inappropriate as a secondary reconstructive procedure for patients who have failed to acquire esophageal voice.

THE CLASSICAL INDICATION for total laryngectomy is squamous cell carcinoma of the larynx with rigid fixation of the glottis. In the majority of instances, patients with fixed T3 laryngeal carcinoma originating at the glottic, the supraglottic, or even the subglottic levels will be found suitable for a slightly less extensive resection. A small segment of uninvolved larynx (conventionally sacrificed in total laryngectomy) can be spared with adequate tumor-free margins. It cannot be reconstituted to allow breathing, but it can be readily incorporated into a tracheopharyngeal shunt suitable for the production of voice.

The advantage of constructing a speaking shunt that incorporates a preserved innervated myomucosal laryngeal remnant is that the resulting fistula will contract during swallowing. These contractions offer reliable resistance to the problem of aspiration, which has hitherto restricted the applicability of vocal reconstructive surgery.

CONVENTIONAL TREATMENT OF T3 AND T4 LARYNGEAL CANCER

Total laryngectomy is widely favored because of its high cure rate in experienced hands. This has been felt to justify its major drawback—loss of the voice. The significance of this devastating complication, which is well appreciated by surgeons who advise total laryngectomy, has lead to three types of rehabilitative management plans. In one widely held approach, laryngectomy is not applied until and unless a full course of radiotherapy has proven unsuccessful. In the second, surgery is performed with efforts directed toward early intensive postlaryngectomy speech therapy aimed at producing esophageal voice or skillful use of an artificial larynx. In the third, primary or secondary attempts at surgical vocal reconstruction are attempted.

Hawkins (1975) reviewed the results of radiotherapy for a large series of T₃ glottic cancer patients treated at a radiotherapy center: two out of ten patients remained alive and kept their larynx when this approach was followed; two more required a total laryngectomy to survive; two of ten died of other causes; and four of ten died of uncontrolled laryngeal cancer when recurrences (local, regional, or systemic) proved unamenable to secondary treatment.

If 80 percent of patients die, undergo laryngectomy, or both when radiation is relied upon as the initial treatment, laryngectomy will remain an important primary alternative. Sixty-five percent of patients reviewed by DeSanto (1977) were cured by this operation alone. Thus the patients could enter speech-therapy programs immediately without the postoperative morbidity and delays that frequently follow surgical salvage of radiation failure, and more than half these patients achieved satisfactory esophageal voice. On the other hand, the American Cancer Society study (Horn 1962) showed that one-third of laryngectomees responding to a poll were unable to utilize esophageal speech and were forced to rely on handwriting or electromechanical aids.

The third option—creation of a tracheopharyngeal fistula—encompasses a long history and a great number of modifications, including laryngeal transplantation and implantation of prosthetic larynges. Of all the rehabilitative approaches, in only one instance has an attempt at laryngeal transplantation been reported and in a patient whose original lesion was not T₃. The patient died with a parastomal recurrence within one year. A handful of attempts at extrapharyngeal electronic implants have been attempted with variable success, as problems of power supply and voluntary control have been hard to overcome. The creation of an internal tracheopharyngeal fistula has now commanded the attention of many surgeons.

FISTULA SPEECH

The observation that voice can reliably be restored by simply connecting the airway to the foodway after laryngectomy has been known since the first laryngectomy in 1873. Because of the associated complications (aspiration and pneumonia), attempts at maintaining such a connection were generally abandoned by laryngologists by the early part of the twentieth century. The subject was reopened periodically thereafter; in the 1960s its modern renaissance may be said to have occurred. So many procedures have been proposed and described in the last twenty years that one hesitates to add another. The very number attests to the fact that none have been found totally satisfactory.

On the other hand, anecdotal cases have often provided spectacular results. These have inspired inevitable attempts to repeat or improve upon observable successes. Some fistulas came to rely on staged reconstruction in the anterior neck through the use of skin flaps and skin grafts to control aspiration. Attempts to valve the tubes by angling their entry into the pharynx or kinking them with a regional muscular sling were also reported. Some success was achieved when the airway and foodway were connected externally by means of a valved mechanical appliance. The simplest procedures have been those that utilize a short, internal, mucosal-lined tracheopharyngeal shunt; however, sizes and shapes of the shunts have been critical in these procedures. Thoughtful surgeons continue to question the indications, safety, and reproducability of these procedures. Many patients with fistulas of sufficient caliber to permit speech are also prone to aspiration. The small size of the fistula or tortuous course to prevent aspiration often does not allow for speech.

PERSONAL EXPERIENCE

We have attempted to combine the modality having the best local cancer control rate (primary surgery) with the simplest reconstructive speaking mechanism (an internal mucosal-lined fistula in which no appliance is used). We avoid aspiration by creating a flaccid tube that constricts during swallowing because of recurrent laryngeal nerve innervation of the remnant of the vocalis, cricoarytenoids, and thyroarytenoid on the nontumor-bearing segment of the larynx. We avoid stenosis by preserving a small, continuous band of mucosa from the trachea to the hypopharynx. Adequate dimensions for low-pressure speech are achieved by augmenting the mucosal lining with a simple, inferiorly based hypopharyngeal flap. Our procedure does not destroy the patient's ability to learn esophageal speech should that option be required. It adds about thirty minutes to the operating time over a conventional total laryngectomy. It has also been found applicable in T3 carcinoma of the glottic, supraglottic, and subglottic levels, though it is not suitable for patients who have previously had a total laryngectomy. We also do not feel that it is safe in postirradiated patients who have clinically indistinct tumor margins. Only those patients with a safe band of tumor-free endolarynx that can be identified, isolated, and preserved and is innervated are suitable candidates. Fortunately, most laryngeal cancers involve one side and the front of the larynx. The segment we seek to preserve, and its innervation, are contralateral and posterior. More T3 cases are suitable for this operation than are not. Naturally, the occasional case in which an even more limited procedure can be done, such as a hemilaryngectomy, is excluded, since our operation commits the patient to a permanent tracheostomy.

Our first case was operated on in 1974, and ten consecutive cases form the subject of this report. To date (June 1980) there have been no significant instances of stenosis, nor has there been recurrence of cancer. Each patient in the series speaks intelligibly, and in no case has a patient required termination of the connection or revision surgery because of aspiration.

TECHNIQUE

The detailed technique of our procedure (Pearson 1980) has been reported at the 1980 Western Section Triologic Meeting and is summarized here.

The extent and pathology of the lesion are confirmed by careful office examination and subsequent preliminary laryngoscopy at the time of the operation. The point of entry into the subglottis is determined at the laryngoscopy and the fact that this area is free from cancer is established. The extent of involvement of the true vocal cord on the uninvolved side is carefully recorded so that the amount of true cord to be preserved on the uninvolved side can be judged with accuracy. The degree of involvement of the supraglottic airway and the margin that can be selected through the uninvolved false cord is accurately determined.

A permanent tracheotomy is created through the fourth tracheal ring, and the anesthetic tubing is removed to this location.

A neck dissection is usually indicated in extensive laryngeal cancers, and this is carried out through an appropriate cervical incision. The neck-dissection specimen can be removed from the larynx in a continuous fashion, and the accessory nerve can almost always be preserved safely. The discontinuous neck dissection provides good access to the larynx, and preservation of the accessory nerve greatly reduces the shoulder morbidity, which is otherwise associated with neck dissection.

The larynx is exposed in the neck, and the narrow vascular pedicles and strap muscles are divided on the tumor-bearing side exactly as they would be in a conventional total laryngectomy (*see* Fig. 14-1). The adjacent soft tissues and ipsilateral thyroid lobe and isthmus are mobilized to be included with the laryngectomy specimen. The strap muscles are mobilized off the contralateral side of the larynx, and the cricothyroid triangle (whose borders are the cricothyroid muscle, the thyroid cartilage, and the cricothyroid ligament) is clearly identified. The thyroid cartilage and hyoid bone are divided vertically on the uninvolved side. The laryngeal ventricle is penetrated with a scalpel, and an offside vertical laryngotomy is gradually developed from below moving upwards. An exact appreciation of how this cut enters the larynx is essential for the laryngotomy to be developed with safety. Erroneous placement too close to the midline risks inadequate tumor resection. Conversely, posterior displacement will sacrifice the endolaryngeal segment one hopes to preserve. (*see* Fig. 14-2)

The margins of the laryngotomy are spread with hooks, and the vallecula is transected at the same level as would be appropriate in a total laryngectomy. This greatly improves visualization of the endolaryngeal soft tissues and allows the laryngotomy to be extended inferiorly to include the vocal cord, the cricoid and, if necessary, the upper trachea on the involved side. If the laryngotomy discloses that the lower margin of the cricoid can be preserved and a hemilaryngectomy will be adequate, the procedure can be downgraded to this less-extensive resection. On the other hand, if the need for a total laryngectomy is revealed, it can be revised upwards by abandoning the laryngotomy and continuing as a conventional laryngectomy. We have not encountered the need for such conversion, but the operative sequence admits these possibilities. (*see* Fig. 14-3)

The posterior endolarynx is exposed through the laryngotomy, and the line of resection on the posterior cricoid plate is chosen and executed. The cut extends through the mucosa and the entire height of the posterior cricoid plate in the midline. This destroys the rigidity of the larynx and allows it to be opened like a book. The inferior line of resection in the trachea is connected to the lower end of the posterior cricoid division. The larynx is dissected from the postlaryngeal soft tissues. The aryepiglottic fold and ipsilateral pyriform fossa, now on the stretch, are divided with appropriate attention to the maintenance of adequate tumor margins. Thus the specimen is delivered (*see* Figure 14-4).

The adequacy of the surgical margins are verified by experienced quick-section histopathologic examination. This examination is critical.

When it is certain the margins are clear, an uninvolved strip of mucosa is left, thus connecting the upper trachea to the pharynx. This strip is simply the remnant of trachea, subglottis, true vocal cord, arytenoid and posterior false cord and aryepiglottic fold of the uninvolved side. The recurrent laryngeal nerve, which enters the larynx behind the cricothyroid joint on this side, reaches the segment behind the residual cricoid remnant. The superior laryngeal nerve also remains intact.

This innervated endolaryngeal tissue is now used to fashion a flaccid phonatory shunt. Because the shunt will be soft-walled, a permanent tracheostomy will need to be retained. The remaining cricoid cartilage remnant (which prevents the myomucosal strip from being tubed) is resected, except for the important cartilage in the immediate vicinity of the recurrent laryngeal nerve. The

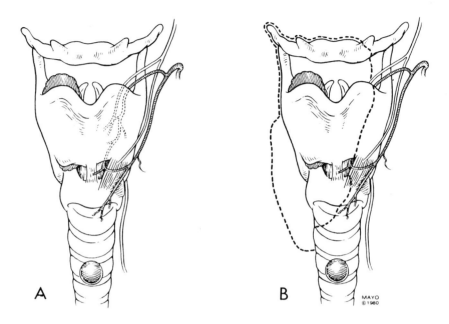

Figure 14-1. (*A*) Extent of resection in extended hemilaryngectomy. (*B*) Larynx, omitting epiglottis for clarity. Tumor on right side. Neurovascular anatomy on the left side. Reproduced with permission from the *Laryngoscope*, *90* (12), December, 1980.

residual thyroid lamina is also discarded. The myomucosal strip can now be tubed, but the diameter of the tube should first be augmented by turning down an inferiorly based, full-thickness mucosal flap from the opposite cut margin of the pharyngotomy. This, of course, is only possible if sufficient pharynx remains (*see* Figure 14-5). When this flap is turned downward, its tip meets the cut edge of the trachea, and its medial margin can be united to the endolaryngeal myomucosal strip (*see* Figure 14-6). Tubing of the shunt is now achieved by closing the lateral edge of the pharyngeal flap to the anterior edge of the preserved endolaryngeal strip. If this closure is carried out from below moving upwards, a point is reached at which nothing remains to be closed but a conventional postlaryngecomy pharyngotomy (*see* Figure 14-7). This too is completed, the neck wound is closed, and a tracheotomy tube is installed, along with appropriate drains and

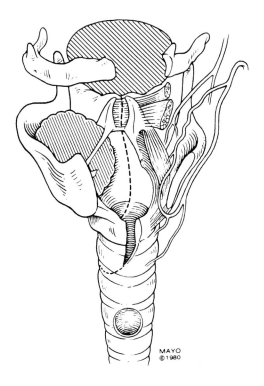

Figure 14-2. Schematic view of the lateral thyrotomy on the left side. Note the transglottic tumor on the right side. Reproduced with permission from the *Laryngoscope, 90* (12), December, 1980.

dressings, as in a total laryngectomy and neck dissection (*see* Figures 14-8, 14-9, and 14-10).

RESULTS

Data on the first ten consecutive cases are charted in Table 14-1. Eight patients had T₃ squamous cell carcinomas of the larynx, one patient had a large cricoid chondrosarcoma, and one patient had a primary squamous cell carcinoma of the right pyriform fossa. The intrinsic laryngeal cases include three glottic, two transglottic, two subglottic, and one supraglottic lesion. Of seven

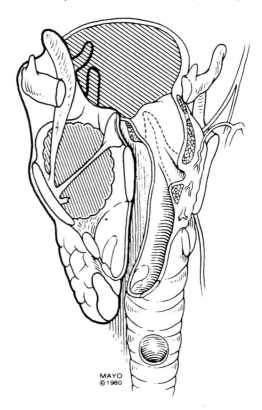

Figure 14-3. After the lateral thyrotomy, the posterior intralaryngeal cut is made. Hemilaryngectomy specimen is shown on the left side (patient's right). Reproduced with permission from the *Laryngoscope, 90*(12), December, 1980.

neck dissections performed in association with the primary laryngeal surgery, only two revealed histologically positive nodes. The duration of follow-up remains too short to assume that the cure rate is identical to that of total laryngectomy. On the other hand, intraoperative visualization is improved over that achieved during laryngectomy, and the negative histologic margins are more generous than those commonly accepted in supraglottic laryngectomy operations.

One of us (D.E. Hartman) has measured the subglottic pressures for five isolated vowels and eight consonant-vowel combinations for each of these patients two months postopera-

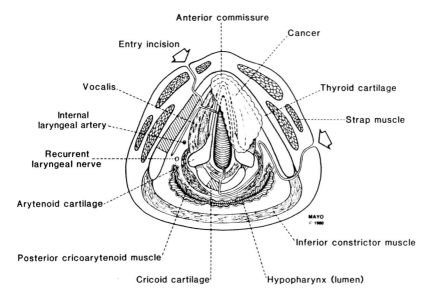

Figure 14-4. This is a cross section to show the extent of resection. Note the inclusion of cricoid. Reproduced with permission from the *Laryngoscope*, *90*(12), December, 1980.

tive in order to establish the opening pressures and those used at the time of speech. The airway pressures required for voice ranged from approximately 16 to 95 cm of water. Cough pressures exceeded this range. Opening pressures average approximately 10 cm below those used in conversational voice.

Speech therapy has been particularly useful in encouraging automatic and synchronous valving of the tracheal stoma with the finger of choice. Precise articulation of speech sounds, reduction of the speaking rate, and appropriate phrasing are refined with a speech pathologist's help. Speech therapy has averaged 3.5 hours for each patient.

Postoperative visualization of the fistula by office mirror examination reveals that the hoped-for sphincteric movement is present. The average hospitalization of thirteen days compares favorably to that associated with total laryngectomy. In no instance has any significant operative complication been attributable to the creation of the fistula (*see* Table 14-1).

TABLE 14-I.

PATIENT	AGE	SEX	LESION	FOLLOW-UP	*SATISFACTORY FISTULA SPEECH
1.	69	F	T₃ GLOTTIC GR. II SCE	6 Yr., 7 Mo.	Yes
2.	62	M	T₃ SUPRAGLOTTIC GR. II SCE	3 Yr., 5 Mo.	Yes
3.	58	M	T₃ GLOTTIC GR. II SCE	2 Yr., 1 Mo.	Yes
4.	63	M	T₃ GLOTTIC GR. II SCE	2 Yr.	Yes
5.	61	M	T₃ TRANSGLOTTIC GR. III SCE	1 Yr. 10 Mo.	Yes
6.	69	M	T₃ SUBGLOTTIC GR. II SCE	1 Yr. 9 Mo.	Yes
7.	68	M	T₃ GLOTTIC GR. II SCE	1 Yr. 8 Mo.	Yes
8.	67	M	T₃ TRANSGLOTTIC GR. II SCE	1 Yr. 7 Mo.	Yes
9.	58	M	T₃ PYRIFORM GR. III SCE	1 Yr. 7 Mo.	Yes
10.	78	M	SUBGLOTTIC CHONDROSARCOMA	1 Yr. 7 Mo.	Yes

*Used by patient in preference to any other mode of communication, readily intelligible to new acquaintance judged superior to esophageal speech by the examining laryngologists.

Table 14-I continued.

SUBGLOTTIC PRESSURES		FISTULA RELATED DEFICIENCIES	COMMENTS
Opening	Conversation		
Not Measured	36.13	1. Initially too tightly closed. Learned esophageal voice	Postoperational wound infection. Pre-operational irradiation. Much prefers her good fistula speech to esophageal
19.12	46.03	2. None	Continues to wear a stomal button to facilitate finger placement
Not Measured	62.98	3. None	Used electrolarynx first eight weeks until fistula speech good
Not Measured	52.12	4. None	Excellent voice, used on radio
Not Measured	16.08	5. Asymptomatic fluid aspiration revealed on barium swallow	Can whistle, as well as speak
25.72	44.00	6. Some asymptomatic aspiration observed with dye	Required special instruction to learn valving
27.38	42.98	7. Initially too tightly closed to voice easily	Gradually loosened voice now excellent
30.46	51.78	8. Slight aspiration on barium swallow. Tolerated without difficulty, cough or restriction of diet	Bulky lesion, initially presenting with stridor
95.10	95.10	9. High-pitched voice	Irradiated (5000 R/5 weeks) Post-operational without damage to fistula
27.42	35.03	10. None	Not squamous cell epithelioma but massive obstructing cricoid sarcoma

**In cm. of H_2O.

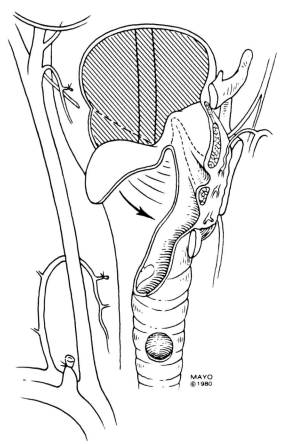

Figure 14-5. Augmentation of the tracheopharyngeal myomucosal strip with the pharyngeal flap. Reproduced with permission from the *Laryngoscope, 90*(12), December, 1980.

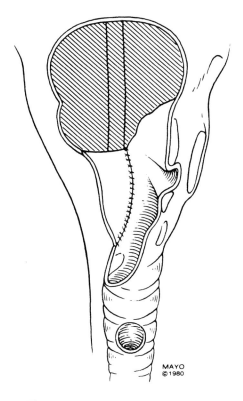

Figure 14-6. The elements of the composite (pharyngeal plus laryngeal) shunt have been approximated and is ready for tubing. Reproduced with permission from the *Laryngoscope, 90*(12), December, 1980.

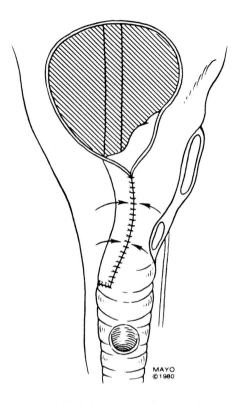

Figure 14-7. The composite shunt shown tubed. Reproduced with permission from the *Laryngoscope*, *90*(12), December, 1980.

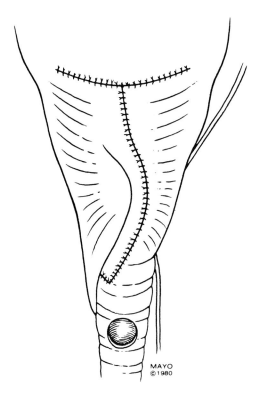

Figure 14-8. The composite shunt is completed and the pharyngotomy closed. Reproduced with permission from the *Laryngoscope, 90*(12), December, 1980.

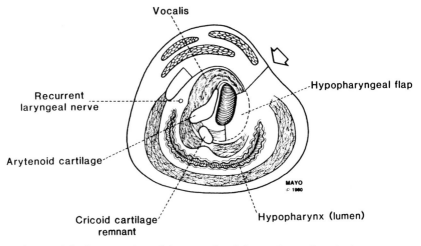

Figure 14-9. Cross section of the completed shunt. Reproduced with permission from the *Laryngoscope, 90*(12), December, 1980.

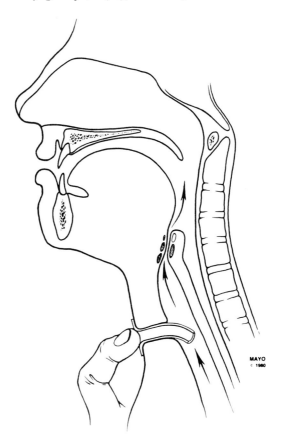

Figure 14-10. The mechanism of speech production after extended hemilaryngectomy and composite shunt. Reproduced with permission from the *Laryngoscope, 90*(12), December, 1980.

REFERENCES

Hawkins, N.V.: The treatment of glottic carcinoma: an analysis of 800 cases. *Laryngoscope, 85*:1485-1493, 1975.

DeSanto, L.W., Devine, K.D., and Lillie, J.C.: Cancer of the larynx: glottic cancer. Surg Clin North Am 57:611-620, 1977.

Horn, D.: *Laryngectomy Survey Report.* Eleventh Annual Meeting, International Association of Laryngectomees, Memphis, Tennessee, 1962.

Pearson, B.W., Woods, R.D., and Hartman, D.E.: Extended hemilaryngectomy for T3 glottic carcinoma with preservation of speech and swallowing. *Laryngoscope, 90*:1950-1961, 1980.

NEOGLOTTIC RECONSTRUCTION: THE STAFFIERI TECHNIQUE

BYRON J. BAILEY, BRUCE LEIPZIG AND CERI M. GRIFFITHS

ABSTRACT

This presentation reviews the historical evolution of surgical procedures designed to restore vocal function following total laryngectomy, with emphasis on the technique of neoglottic reconstruction developed by Mario Staffieri. The goal of this group of surgical procedures is the development of a one-way, tracheopharyngeal fistula that permits the passage of pulmonary air in a manner that generates a vibrating airstream comparable to that produced by the normal larynx. The prevention of salivary and food aspiration is an essential characteristic of successful neoglottic reconstruction. The Staffieri technique is a one-stage operation that appears to be the most satisfactory operation used for this purpose at the present time. The complications that must be avoided with neoglottic reconstruction are (1) long-term stenosis postoperatively, (2) stenosis of the fistula with postoperative radiation therapy, (3) compromise of the surgical removal of the cancer, and (4) an unacceptable degree of aspiration. Observations will be made concerning the quality and intelligibility of neoglottic speech, the surgical success rate, and the complications associated with our patient experience.

INTRODUCTION

THE QUEST FOR METHODS to restore speech following the loss of the larynx dates back to the middle of the nineteenth century. Since the first report of successful esophageal speech by Reynaud (Arnold 1960) in 1841, many physicians have pursued ingenious avenues in their quest for a better solution. As society has become more complex, the need for effective verbal communication has grown. The social, economic, and psychological impact of laryngectomy is staggering, and conversely, measures that can restore effective communication are of immeasurable value to the victim of cancer or trauma and to the family of the victim.

The surgical removal of the entire larynx eliminates the power source for vocalization. In our personal experience, this loss has been crippling to many of our patients who are unable to read or write or who may live in remote regions of the state where speech therapy is not available.

In the Department of Otolaryngology at the University of Texas Medical Branch in Galveston, a surgical technique for reconstruction of a neoglottis, or pseudoglottis, has been utilized to re-establish a power source for vocalization. The technique that has been employed at UTMB is based on a surgical procedure reported by Staffieri et al. (1976) in 1970. The initial results were very encouraging and, while our enthusiasm is somewhat tempered with the passage of more time, it does appear that there is a place for this operation in the field of rehabilitative surgery until better methods become available.

The objective of this surgical procedure, and similar operations, is the development of a one-way, tracheopharyngeal fistula that permits the passage of pulmonary air in a manner so as to generate a vibrating airstream comparable to that produced by the vibrating vocal folds in the normal larynx. The prevention of salivary and food aspiration of a significant degree is an essential characteristic of successful neoglottic reconstruction. The Staffieri technique is a one-stage operation that appears to be the most satisfactory operation available for this purpose at the present time.

It is the purpose of this chapter to review the historical evolution of this technique, to describe the nature of the surgical procedure, and to report our observations in the terms of vocal function and postoperative complications. The procedure of Staffieri appears to be an acceptable form of neoglottic reconstruction in that it is reported to have the greatest success in avoiding (1) long-term postoperative stenosis, (2) stenosis of the fistula with postoperative radiation therapy, (3) compromise of the surgical removal of the cancer, and (4) an unacceptable degree of aspiration.

HISTORICAL REVIEW

The years between 1859 and 1942 were filled with reports* of creative efforts to design and implement surgical procedures and prosthetic devices that would be of assistance to the laryngectomized patient; these are summarized for the reader in Table 15-I. Unfortunately, the limitations of surgical and mechanical technology during those years presented major obstacles that could only be overcome with partial success. These reports consistently refer to a very small number of patients, as a rule, and leave the reader with an opinion that the problems were of such magnitude that the efforts were ultimately abandoned.

However, by contrast, the work of Briani (1952) between 1942 and 1952 appears to have heralded the opening of a modern era of surgical procedures and prosthetic devices with which we are rapidly gaining experience today. Briani was an innovative Italian surgeon who developed a functional, external air-bypass prosthesis that could be fitted into a surgically created, skin-lined, cervical-esophageal fistula. The basic conceptualization that he employed has been carried in many directions by others over the past three decades.

Working independently in this country, Conley has reported his experiences with both external and internal tracheopharyngeal shunts in reports published in 1958 (Conley, DeAmesti, and Pierce 1958) and 1969 (Conley 1969). Conley's important contributions were followed quickly by reports from various head and neck surgeons in North America and Great Britain. Some of the most widely accepted and utilized surgical procedures have been those described by Asai (1972), Montgomery and Toohill (1968), Montgomery (1972), Edwards (1975), Taub and Bergner (1973), Taub (1974), Sisson et al. (1975), and, most recently, Singer and Blom (1980).

---

*For a listing of these reports, see Asai 1972; Briani 1952; Brown 1925; Calcaterra 1971; Conley 1969; Edwards 1975; Goode 1975; Guttman 1935; Hanson 1940; Kitamura 1970; Komorn 1973, 1974; McGrail 1971; Montgomery 1968, 1972; Rodgers 1975; Shedd 1974, 1975; Sisson 1975; Taub 1973, 1974.

TABLE 15-I. Speech Rehabilitation After Total Laryngectomy:
Chronology of Developments

Date	Scientist	Development
1841	Reynaud described esophageal speech, followed by reports by Bourquet (1856), Sawyer (1856), and Bose (1865).	
1859	Czermak developed a reed-containing tube which passed externally from the trachea to the mouth.	
1861	Bruns developed a flexible metal tube (containing a rubber band) that was placed externally between the trachea and mouth.	
1874	Gussenbauer developed a tracheopharyngeal air bypass prosthesis with a reed that required a pharyngeal fistula.	
1887	Stoerk devised a tracheooral tube with a whistle held between the teeth. It was later modified to be powered by a hand-held bellows.	
1925	Brown reported the use of a pitch whistle and ear speculum inserted into a small pharyngeal fistula.	
1927	Beck presented a patient who had created a tracheopharyngeal fistula with an ice pick and had developed speech.	
1928	Scuri described a patient with speech after the spontaneous development of a tracheopharyngeal fistula.	
1935	Guttman reported three patients who had been able to speak following a tracheopharyngeal fistula created by a diathermy knife.	
1942-1958	Briani developed and reported speech rehabilitation employing a skin-lined, cervical-esophageal fistula and an external air bypass prosthesis.	
1958-1959	Conley developed external and internal tracheoesophageal fistula techniques.	
1962	Ogura, et al. described an experimental technique (in dogs) for creation of a tracheopharyngeal fistula.	
1965	Asai described a staged technique for creation of a tracheopharyngeal internal voice tunnel.	
1965	Barton reported a tracheooral speech tunnel technique.	
1968	Montgomery and Toohill developed tracheoesophageal and tracheopharyngeal fistula techniques.	
1969	Goode published his work on an external electronic laryngeal prosthesis that utilized a pharyngeal fistula.	
1970-1971	McGrail and Oldfield reported the use of a deltopectoral flap to create a tracheopharyngeal fistula for speech.	
1970	Kitamura described a tracheopharyngeal fistula for speech rehabilitation.	
1971	Calcaterra reported his findings involving a tracheoesophageal fistula for speech.	
1972	Shedd developed an external reed-fistula prosthesis, which utilizes a pharyngocutaneous fistula.	
1973	Komorn published his experience with a tracheoesophageal fistula technique.	
1973	Edwards described another form of tracheopharyngeal shunt using an air bypass prosthesis.	
1973	Taub reported his work with an esophageal fistula and an external air bypass prosthesis.	
1974	Shedd developed a second air bypass prosthesis which employs a higher pharyngeal fistula.	
1975	Sisson and McConnel published their technique which uses an external air	

Table 15-I continued.

	bypass prosthesis and a pharyngeal fistula.
1975	Rogers, Frederickson, and Bryce described an implanted electronic laryngeal prosthesis that had been studied experimentally in dogs.

Reproduced with permission from the *Annals of Otology, Rhinology, and Laryngology,* *85*(4):472, 1976.
Reproduced with permission from the *Laryngoscope, 81*(11):1742-1771, 1971.

Table 15-II. Noninvasive Air-Powered Methods of Vocal Rehabilitation

	Air Source	Vibrator
Esophageal speech	Esophageal reservoir	Pharyngeal mucosa
Czermak's device	Pulmonary air	Rubber band
Bruns' device	Pulmonary air	Rubber band
Stoerk's device	Mechanical bellows	Whistle
Tokyo device	Pulmonary air	Rubber band

Reproduced with permission from the *Annals of Otology, Rhinology and Laryngology,* *85*(4):472, 1976.

During the past ten years there has been a virtual explosion of diverse ideas for mechanical, electronic, and surgical methods that show promise for expanding the spectrum of solutions to this complex problem. In order to attempt to place the neoglottic reconstructive surgical procedures into context in this field, we should view it in terms of a classification system. Table 15-II (Nelson, Parkin, and Potter 1975; Miller 1971; Goode 1975; Bailey and Goode 1975; Bailey, Griffiths, and Everett 1976) presents the noninvasive, air-powered methods for vocal rehabilitation after total laryngectomy. After each, we show the source for the air column and the vibrating component.

In Table 15-III the invasive procedures for pulmonary air-powered rehabilitation are shown. This table notes after each technique such variables as the requirement for a prosthesis, location of the fistula, and the presumed vibrating source.

The most recent entries into the field have been electronic devices, some of which are external and others are for internal implantation. In Table 15-IV, the various electronically powered devices for vocal rehabilitation are listed.

And so it is possible to trace a rich history that has evolved slowly at first and then much more rapidly in recent years.

Table 15-III. Invasive Procedures for Pulmonary Air-Powered
Vocal Rehabilitation

	Prosthesis Required	External Fistula/ Internal Shunt	Fistula/ Shunt Location	Presumed Vibrator Sound Source
Conley-I	No	I	T-E	M & T
Conley-II	Yes	E	T-E	M & T
Montgomery-I	Yes	E	E-E	M & T
Calcaterra	No	I	T-E	M & T
Komorn	No	I	T-E	M & T
Taub	Yes	E	T-E (? low pharyngeal)	M
Gussenbauer	Yes	E	T-P (H)	Reed
Brown	Yes	E	T-P (L)	Pitch Whistle
Guttman	No	I	T-P (L)	M & T
Briani	Yes	E	T-P (H)	M
Asai	No	I	T-P (H)	T
Montgomery	Yes/No	E	T-P (L)	M
McGrail	Yes	I	T-P (H)	T
Kitamura	No	I	T-P (H)	T
Shedd-I	Yes	E	T-P (L)	Reed
Shedd-II	Yes	E	T-P (H)	M
Edwards	Yes	E	T-P (H)	T
Sisson	Yes	E	T-P (H)	T O
Barton	Yes	I	T-Oral	T O
Staffieri	No	I	T-E	M

E—External. I—Internal. T-E—Tracheoesophageal. T-P—Tracheopharyngeal.
(H)—High. (L)—Low. M—Mucosa. T—Tunnel. T O—Tunnel Opening.
Reproduced with permission from the *Annals of Otology, Rhinology and Laryngology*,
85(4):472, 1976.

Table 15-IV. Electronic-Powered Devices for
Vocal Rehabilitation

	Varieties of Devices
External transoral	(Cooper-Rand, Tait, Ticchioni pipe)
External transcervical	(Aurex, Kett, Electro-larynx)
Goode	External sound source—Pharyngocutaneous fistula
Pichler	Intraoral (dental) transducer with wireless transduction
Frederickson	Implanted pharyngeal transducer with wireless transduction
Bailey	Implanted pharyngeal transducer with wireless transduction

Reproduced with permission from the *Annals of Otology, Rhinology and Laryngology*,
85(4):472, 1976.

However, between the lines of these publications—rich in innovation and creative thinking—runs a persistent thread of partial success, frequent failure, and frustration in efforts to find a reliable and ideal solution to the rehabilitation of the laryngectomized patient. There does seem to be a clear reason for an optimistic perception of the future. It also seems that it is time to think in terms of a hierarchy of solutions. For instance, the most desirable rehabilitative options would be those in which speech can be restored without the wearing of a prosthesis or the use of external or implantable devices. The author prefers to call this group of solutions Level 1 (most desirable). The Staffieri technique, when successful, is a Level 1 solution that can be accomplished frequently as a one-stage surgical procedure free of major postoperative complications and not requiring significant postoperative care above and beyond that which is standard for a total laryngectomy for cancer.

Level 2 solutions would be that group of techniques and devices in which a very simple surgical procedure might be employed and a very convenient prosthesis might be required for successful vocal rehabilitation. The surgical technique of hypopharyngeal puncture and the simple plastic tube/valve being popularized by Singer and Blom (1980) would be an excellent example of a Level 2 rehabilitative solution.

Level 3 rehabilitative strategies would include those requiring a major surgical procedure (such as the creation of an extensive tracheoesophageal fistula), the wearing of a complex or bulky prosthetic device, or the implantation of a prosthetic device. The current models of air-bypass prostheses or an implanted electronic laryngeal prosthesis would be examples of Level 3 rehabilitative strategies.

When viewed in this manner, it becomes desirable to place a premium on the most effective means for rehabilitation that can be found in Level 1 strategies. Of course, esophageal speech is also a Level 1 rehabilitative technique; therefore, it is necessary to quantify the degree to which the patient is able to function and the limitations that are imposed by the particular strategy that has been selected. If there is a lack of success or lack of satisfaction with Level 1 solutions, it would be reasonable to proceed with the next level and to continue to do so until the patient can return to society and to the family with appropriate communication skills.

THE TECHNIQUE OF NEOGLOTTIC RECONSTRUCTION

A total laryngectomy is performed in a manner that would be considered appropriate for the size and location of the carcinoma. As a rule, the patient would have an extensive tumor that was felt to be inappropriate for a conservation, partial-laryngectomy technique or for radiation therapy. Usually, a wide-field laryngectomy is performed along with a radical neck dissection, and in most cases, the procedure will be followed by radiation therapy after healing has been completed.

The only modification from standard, total-laryngectomy surgery is made to accommodate the construction of the neoglottis, and adequate cancer surgery is never compromised, even if it would make it impossible for a neoglottic reconstruction to be performed.

The trachea is transected below the level of the cricoid cartilage, and the incision is beveled inferiorly from the anterior margin of the trachea to the posterior (soft tissue) wall of the trachea. This will be the angled, recipient site for the neoglottic flap (*see* Fig. 15-1). The purpose of the bevelling step is to create an inclined plane for the surface in which the neoglottic fistula is located. This maneuver appears to eliminate the presence of a bubbling quality to the voice that has been described when the tracheal transection is horizontal. The surgical dissection begins between the posterior tracheal wall and the anterior esophageal wall and is continued cranially in order to develop a flap of post-cricoid muscle and mucosa that is to be used in the reconstruction. When this dissection has been completed, the hypopharynx is entered at the geometric site located at the greatest distance from the margin of the carcinoma. The point of entry into the hypopharynx is then developed and extended to outline the cephalic or superior-most portion of the myomucosal flap utilized in the neoglottic reconstruction.

A permanent tracheostoma is created with an approximate diameter of two centimeters by resection of the skin overlying the

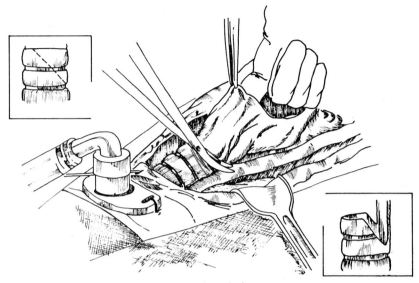

Tracheal ring beveled...

Figure 15-1. The larynx has been separated from the trachea between the cricoid cartilage and the first tracheal ring. A second cut is made to bevel the end of the tracheal stump. Reproduced with permission from the *Annals of Otology, Rhinology and Laryngology, 89*:204-208, 1980.

anterior tracheal wall at the level of the third or fourth tracheal ring. It is sometimes possible to create the stoma at a lower level if further tracheal resection is required. In some cases, neoglottic reconstruction has been accomplished at the same level as the standard tracheostoma (located at the uppermost end of the trachea). In the event that an extremely low tracheostoma is created, it is helpful to stabilize the trachea by means of an anchoring suture placed between the trachea and the periosteum of the superior margin of the sternum. Meticulous approximation of the cut-skin edges to the tracheal mucosa is of considerable, technical importance. With careful construction of the stoma, the healing will permit fitting with a tracheal button after the wound has healed. This is very helpful in terms of patient convenience, as it permits closure of the stoma by a fingertip when talking and also could provide an airtight seal for any valved prosthesis that might be employed in the future.

The surgeon's attention is then directed to the myomucosal flap and the posterior wall (soft tissue) of the trachea, which should be sutured to the esophageal wall in order to maintain stability and a constant relationship between these two layers. This will aid in the accurate positioning of the neoglottis and will avoid dislocation of the neoglottic site secondary to a migration of the flap during the healing period. This will also permit the surgeon to place a slight amount of tension on the flap in the anterioposterior dimension. The flap is then sutured over the top of the tracheal stump, and the surgeon carefully positions and marks the point at which the neoglottis is to be created. This site is located five millimeters posterior to the inner lip of the anterior wall of the trachea. With a sharp-pointed scalpel blade (No. 11 blade), an incision is made through the muscle and submucosa until the mucous membrane of the adjacent esophagus can be seen. The incision is approximately five millimeters long. This step is facilitated by placing the gloved finger into the lumen of the upper-cervical esophagus, as shown in Figure 15-2.

The intact mucosa of the cervical esophagus is then grasped through this small incision and drawn outward toward the surgeon between the delicate muscle fibers. An incision is made through the mucosa, and the mucosa is gently retracted through the opening so that a fistula is formed. The mucosal edges are then stabilized with sutures of 6-0 Dexon®, which are very carefully placed. Care is taken to be certain that only the mucosa (and no submucosa) is included in this suture so that postoperative prolapse of the neoglottic fistula can be avoided, as shown in Figure 15-3. Careful attention to this sort of detail during the surgical procedure itself is felt to be essential if gapping of the fistula is to be avoided. Problems of significant and intolerable aspiration are associated with excessive gapping (openness) of the neoglottic fistula.

Once the neoglottis has been constructed, some surgeons prefer to place a long black silk suture from the tracheostoma through the neoglottis and pharynx and out through the nasal passage. The suture serves a dual purpose in that it can be utilized to identify the neoglottis for postoperative dilation in the operating room

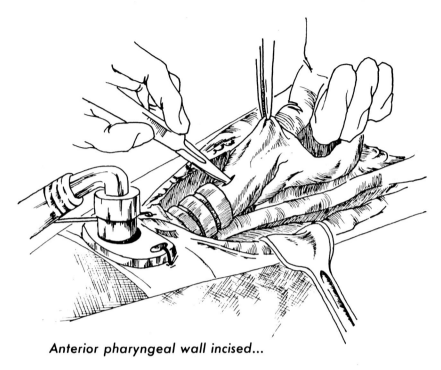

Anterior pharyngeal wall incised...

Figure 15-2. The anterior wall of the hypopharynx-cervical esophagus region is incised to create the "neoglottis" fistula. Reproduced with permission from the *Annals of Otology, Rhinology and Laryngology, 89*:204-208, 1980.

when necessary or it can be used to maintain the patency of the neoglottis during postoperative radiation therapy. Gentle manipulation of the suture does seem to be successful in breaking up the small fibrous adhesions and maintaining the proper function of the neoglottic fistula.

Other surgeons prefer the use of a custom-made silastic obturator that is placed in the neoglottis at the time of surgery and left in place during the first four weeks of healing.

After completing the neoglottic reconstruction, the flap is sutured carefully into position over the superior margin of the tracheal stump as shown in Figure 15-4. This closure is accomplished in two layers by using 3-0 Dexon suture and carefully avoiding any tension laterally on the flap as a further precaution in the avoidance of a tendency for gapping of the neoglottic

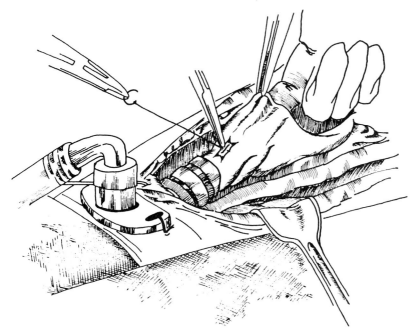

Mucosa sutured to anterior wall...

Figure 15-3. The mucosa is pulled through the opening, incised, and sutured in place. Reproduced with permission from the *Annals of Otology, Rhinology and Laryngology, 89*:204-208, 1980.

fistula. Closure of the hypopharynx and skin and the use of postoperative wound drainage are standard and unmodified from the customary surgical practice of the surgeon.

RESULTS

The experience with the Staffieri technique at the University of Texas Medical Branch in Galveston was associated with an initial enthusiasm that has been modified and tempered as additional observations have been made. In the first report by Griffiths and Love (1978), a success rate of 80 percent was reported. The case histories and details of eight patients were presented, and the authors expressed their feeling that the technique seemed to offer great potential for a number of reasons:

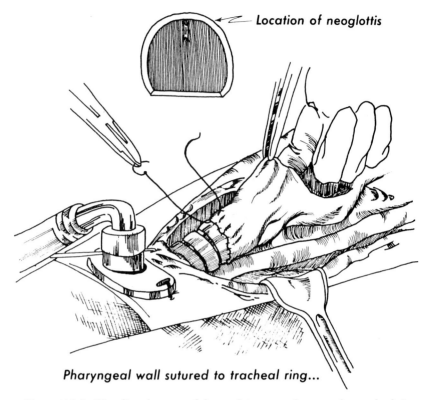

Figure 15-4. The flap is sutured into place over the superior end of the trachea, and the pharyngeal defect is closed. Reproduced with permission from the *Annals of Otology, Rhinology and Laryngology, 89:*204-208, 1980.

1. The neoglottic reconstruction can be accomplished without compromising the surgical resection for cancer.
2. The surgical procedure is simple.
3. This is a one-step procedure in patients who have not received radiation therapy.
4. There are no mechanical prostheses to be worn either externally or internally.
5. The time for vocal rehabilitation is short.
6. It is possible to achieve a relatively long phonation time, which results in much-improved speech intelligibility.

The authors did observe, however, that there are several disadvantages to the procedure:

1. Vocal quality is hoarse.
2. It is necessary for the patient to have a permanent tracheostomy.
3. The use of one hand is required to occlude the tracheostoma during phonation.
4. Problems with aspiration of a minor nature may develop.

In 1979, Griffiths and Leipzig (1980) reported their observations in regard to twenty-six patients who had undergone neoglottic reconstruction at the University of Texas Medical Branch. They noted that while twenty-two patients (84%) were able to phonate in the early postoperative period, only twenty patients (77%) were capable of producing intelligible speech by means of the neoglottis at one year postoperatively. They noted further that only seventeen (65%) of the patients were actually communicating by means of neoglottic speech at the time of the analysis. A surgical revision of the neoglottis was necessary in order to retain or re-establish vocal function in one-third of the patients (7 patients).

It was noted at the time of this analysis that postoperative irradiation was not contraindicated. The patient group that received radiotherapy (17 patients) did not require neoglottic revision as frequently as the patient group (8 patients) who did not receive postoperative radiotherapy.

Aspiration was noted to be a minor problem in the postoperative period with almost every patient, but was only a significant and prolonged problem with eleven patients. Four of the eleven patients required a revision of the surgical procedure in order to achieve satisfactory control of this problem. In the case of one patient, it was necessary to close the neoglottic fistula, and vocal function was lost. Infection occurred postoperatively to a significant degree in three patients. It was possible by means of revision surgery, however, to restore neoglottic voice production in all three.

The authors noted the importance of avoiding a compromise with adequate cancer surgery in regard primarily to the matter of subglottic extension of the primary tumor. Recurrence of carcinoma or persistence of the original malignancy is usually followed by a fatal outcome.

The group of patients capable of neoglottic speech, but electing not to use this for verbal communication, is of particular interest. The basis for this phenomenon is sometimes rooted in a mechanical origin (phonation may not be accomplished easily due to high opening pressure of the fistula) or may be psychological in origin. The association of a deep-seated depression with the need for total laryngectomy and the anxieties associated with a diagnosis of cancer are well known. Patients who avoid neoglottic speech on the basis of their impression that it has a disagreeable quality are often amenable to persistent counselling and can be encouraged to accept this compromise in vocal quality.

In a subsequent analysis of the UTMB experience with neoglottic reconstruction, Leipzig (1980*b*) cautioned that patients with poor pulmonary function may have difficulty employing the neoglottis for speech. This may be on the basis of a low vital capacity with inability to exceed the opening pressure of the neoglottic fistula or may be related to a restricted tidal volume. He also observed that the absence of adequate pulmonary reserve might predispose the patient with aspiration to a terminal pneumonia.

As experience with the technique continued to grow, some additional issues were noted to have relevance. Leipzig noted that reflux of gastric contents—a problem that is not rare in the elderly population—can result in a subsequent aspiration of these contents into the trachea. He also counselled against the tendency to expand the indications for total laryngectomy and neoglottic reconstruction beyond their appropriate place in the therapeutic armamentarium. Laryngeal tumors that can be managed by means of conservative, partial-laryngectomy procedures should not be drawn into efforts to gain experience with the neoglottic reconstruction technique, and conversely, lesions extending subglottically or into the pyriform sinus may present technical problems that tempt the surgeon to push neoglottic reconstruction beyond its limits. This can work to the disadvantage of the patient in terms of an unnecessarily increased morbidity postoperatively, or even to a problem with excessively high numbers of patients with recurrent or persistent carcinoma.

It was noted that when the neoglottic reconstruction is successful, the results in terms of speech intelligibility are excellent and equivalent to the intelligibility of the best esophageal speakers. The emotive quality of the voice is superior, and the phonation time is much longer. The average patient succeeds in gaining neoglottic speech and communicating by thirteen days after the time of laryngectomy and requires only one or two speech-therapy sessions in order to develop this communication ability.

DISCUSSION

As the size of the neoglottic reconstruction patient group has grown, there has been an increasing awareness of the problems, complications, and pitfalls associated with a new surgical procedure.

The most recent analysis by Leipzig (1980*b*) has just been completed and presented. It deals with a population of fifty patients who underwent primary neoglottic reconstruction and nine patients who underwent secondary neoglottic reconstruction more than one year later following the total-laryngectomy procedure. This most recent analysis contains a number of findings that serve to diminish even further the enthusiasm for neoglottic reconstruction as a routine surgical procedure.

Nine patients have been found to have persistent or recurrent carcinoma. Three of these patients have had a local recurrence at the site of the neoglottic fistula and tracheostoma. Each of the three is noted to have been a patient with extension of the laryngeal primary more than one centimeter inferior to the margin of the true vocal cord, and it is suggested that each should have undergone a more extensive resection of the trachea. There are six other patients who developed evidence of metastatic carcinoma subsequent to the time of their original surgical procedure.

The problem with aspiration following neoglottic reconstruction is now being approached in terms of a grading system that defines the parameters of four separate grades of aspiration ranging from "a bubble present on the neoglottic fistula" (Grade 1) to "pneumonia" (Grade 4). Leipzig notes that all patients have some difficulty with aspiration, but that in 40 percent of the patients in this series who underwent primary reconstruction, the degree of aspiration is a potential threat to the patient's life. Among the nine patients who underwent neoglottic reconstruction as a secondary procedure, the degree of aspiration has been even more serious. Six of those nine patients were evaluated as having Grade 3 and Grade 4 aspiration. There have been problems in achieving fistula closure at the neoglottis with revision surgery in this group. Overall, fourteen of the fifty patients who underwent primary neoglottic reconstruction required revision of their fistula for severe aspiration and seven of these required permanent closure. In the group of secondary neoglottic reconstruction (9 patients) six patients were evaluated as having severe aspiration problems. Most of these patients required or elected to have a closure of their neoglottis.

In terms of an evaluation of the success of this procedure, the bottom line is the development of useful communication using the neoglottic fistula. When the patient elects to employ fistula speech for primary communication, the operation can be considered to be a success. If, on the other hand, the patient finds the speech too difficult or unacceptable for any of a variety of reasons, the procedure cannot be considered to have been successful. On this basis, twenty-five of the fifty patients who underwent a primary neoglottic procedure, and four of the nine patients who underwent a secondary procedure, have successful voice production. We can see, therefore, that neoglottic reconstruction would seem to be successful in an overall percentage of just under one-half of these fifty-nine patients.

SUMMARY

The development of a surgical procedure designed to create a one-way fistula between the trachea and the cervical esophagus or hypopharynx has taken a giant leap forward during the last five years in this country. The Staffieri technique, with its numerous modifications, seems to be finding a solid position in the armamentarium of head and neck cancer surgeons.

While the technique cannot be pushed beyond the limits for which it was designed, and while aspiration and stenosis continue to present problems, the success rate is quite reasonable.

Bearing this in mind, when the procedure results in phonation without aspiration, the patient has been very nicely rehabilitated. There should be no need for a long-term, complex procedure to maintain function, and extensive training is not required. No prosthesis must be worn, and the only price to pay is the need to occlude the tracheostoma with one finger to accomplish fistula speech.

The speech that is produced is of excellent quality, can contain emotional subtleties, and provides an excellent phonation time in the presence of adequate pulmonary function. This is an ideal model for Level 1 rehabilitative strategies as referred to previously by this author. Recognizing that we are viewing this technique along the time course of rehabilitative evolution, the next step that comes forward to replace the neoglottic reconstruction procedure will have a rather impressive standard that must be exceeded if it is to supplant this technique.

We recognize that this material has been prepared in an effort to inform nonsurgical, engineering-oriented scientists to one facet of the state of the art of rehabilitative surgical techniques. We hope that this effort has been informative and helpful and hope that it spurs the reader to pursue new and better strategies for the vocal rehabilitation of the laryngectomee.

REFERENCES

Arnold, G.E.: Alleviation of alaryngeal aphonia with the modern artificial larynx: I. Evolution of artificial speech aids and their value for rehabilitation. *Logos,* 3:55-67, 1960.

Asai, R.: Laryngoplasty after total laryngectomy. *Arch Otolaryngol, 95:* 114-119, 1972.

Bailey, B.J., and Goode, R.L.: New and projected procedures and devices for voice rehabilitation after total laryngectomy. *Can J Otolaryngol, 4:*605-609, 1975.

Bailey, B.J., Griffiths, C.M., and Everett, R.: An implanted electronic laryngeal prosthesis. *Ann Otol Rhinol Laryngol,* 85:472-483, 1976.

Briani, A.A.: Riabilitazione fonetica di laringectomizzati a mezzo della corrente aerea espiratoria polmonare. *Arch Ital Otol,* 63:469-475, 1952.

Brown, R.G.: A simple but effective artificial larynx. *J Laryngol Otol, 40:* 793-797, 1925.

Calcaterra, T.C., and Jafek, R.W.: Tracheoesophageal shunt for speech rehabilitation after total laryngectomy. *Arch Otolaryngol, 94*:124-128, 1971.

Conley, J.: Surgical techniques for the vocal rehabilitation of the postlaryngectomized patient. *Trans Am Acad Ophthalmol Otolaryngol, 73*: 288-299, 1969.

Conley, J.J., DeAmesti, F., and Pierce, M.K.: A new surgical technique for the focal rehabilitation of the laryngectomized patient. *Ann Otol Rhinol Laryngol, 67*:655-664, 1958.

Edwards, N.: Post-laryngectomy vocal rehabilitation using expired air and an external fistula method. *Laryngoscope, 85*:690-699, 1975.

Goode, R.L.: Artificial laryngeal devices in postlaryngectomy rehabilitation. *Laryngoscope, 85*:677-689, 1975.

_____: The development of an improved artificial larynx. *Trans Am Acad Ophthalmol Otolaryngol, 73*:279-287, 1969.

Griffiths, C.M., and Leipzig, B.: Surgical restoration of voice after total laryngectomy: Problems, complications and revision surgery. *Proceedings of the Third International Symposium on Plastic and Reconstructive Surgery of the Head and Neck*, New Orleans, April 1979. In press.

Griffiths, C.M., and Love, J.T.: Neoglottic reconstruction: A preliminary report. *Ann Otol Rhinol Laryngol, 87*:180-184, 1978.

Guttman, M.R.: Tracheohypopharyngeal fistulization: a new procedure for speech production in the laryngectomized patient. *Trans 41st Annual Meeting Am Laryngol Rhinol Otol Soc*, 219-226, 1935.

Hanson, W.L.: A new artificial larynx with a historical review. *Ill Med J, 7*: 483-486, 1940.

Kitamura, T., Kaneko, T., Togawa, K., Tokuyi, U., Takashi, K., Akiyoshi, K., Hisashi, A., and Tetsuzo, M.: Supracricoid laryngectomy: a new technique for vocal rehabilitation. *Laryngoscope, 80*:300-308, 1970.

Komorn, R.M.: Vocal rehabilitation in the laryngectomized patient with a tracheoesophageal shunt. *Ann Otol Rhinol Laryngol, 83*:445-451, 1974.

Komorn, R.M., Weycer, J.S., and Sessions, R.B., and Malone, P.E.: Vocal rehabilitation with a tracheoesophageal shunt. *Arch Otolaryngol, 97*:303-305, 1973.

Leipzig, B.: *Neoglottic Reconstruction Following Total Laryngectomy: a reappraisal*. Presented at the Combined Otolaryngological Spring Meetings, April 12-19, 1980*b*, Palm Beach, Florida.

Leipzig, B., Griffiths, C.M., and Shea, J.P.: Neoglottic reconstruction following total laryngectomy: the Galveston experience. *Ann Otol Rhinol Laryngol, 89*:204-208, 1980*a*.

McGrail, J.S., and Oldfield, D.L.: One-stage operation for vocal rehabilitation at laryngectomy. *Trans Am Acad Ophthalmol Otolaryngol, 75*:510-512, 1971.

Miller, A.H.: Four years experience with the Asai technique for vocal rehabilitation for the laryngectomized patient. *J Laryngol, 85*:567-578, 1971.

Montgomery, W.W.: Postlaryngectomy vocal rehabilitation. *Arch Otolaryngol, 95*:76-83, 1972.

Montgomery, W.W., and Toohill, R.J.: Voice rehabilitation after laryngectomy. *Arch Otolaryngol, 88*:499-506, 1968.

Nelson, I.W., Parkin, J.L., and Potter, J.F.: The modified Tokyo larynx: an improved pneumatic speech aid. *Arch Otolaryngol, 101*:107-108, 1975.

Rodgers, J.H., Fredrickson, J.M., and Bryce, D.P.: New techniques for vocal rehabilitation. *Can J Otolaryngol, 4*:595-604, 1975.

Shedd, D., Bakamjian, V., Sako, K., et al.: Further appraisal of reed-fistula speech following pharyngolaryngectomy. *Can J Otolaryngol, 4*:583-587, 1975.

————: Postlaryngectomy speech rehabilitation by a simplified, single-stage surgical method. *Am J Surg, 128*:505-511, 1974.

Singer, M.I., and Blom, E.D.: Tracheoesophageal puncture: a surgical prosthetic method for postlaryngectomy speech restoration. *Third International Symposium on Plastic and Reconstructive Surgery of the Head and Neck*, New Orleans, April 1979. In press.

Sisson, G.A., McConnel, F.M.S., Logemann, J.A., and Yeh, S.: Voice rehabilitation after laryngectomy: results with the use of a hypopharyngeal prosthesis. *Arch Otolaryngol, 101*:178-181, 1975.

Staffieri, M., Serafini, I., Capretti, C., et al.: *La Riabilitazione Chirurgica della Voce e della Respirazione Dopo Laringectomia Totale.* Bologna, Italy, Associazione Otologi Ospedialieki Italini, 1-222, 1976.

Taub, S.: Voice prosthesis for speech restoration laryngectomees. *Trans Am Acad Ophthalmol Otolaryngol, 78*:287-288, 1974.

Taub, S., and Bergner, L.H.: Air bypass voice prosthesis for vocal rehabilitation of laryngectomees. *Am J Surg, 125*:748-756, 1973.

COMMENTARY ON SURGICAL-ENHANCEMENT METHODS

WILBUR JAMES GOULD

Different approaches to voice preservation and restoration by surgical-reconstructive means has been presented in the preceding three chapters. The goal to be achieved is that of adequate vocal communication when surgical extirpation of a malignant tumor in the larynx is required. All agree that the successful removal of malignant tissue should not in any way be compromised in the attempt to achieve this goal. More than in most surgical procedures for cancer, the threat of destruction of voice has a profound psychological effect upon patients. The destruction of communication ability destroys a fundamental human act, that of speech production. Whenever possible, the restoration of this facility should be fast and in the most natural quality possible. When it can be done safely, the procedure should aim at creation of vocalization by natural airway without a required permanent tracheostomy, so that the phonatory act can be performed with the greatest possible projection ability and without the use of a finger for obstruction of the airway in order to create this sound. The quality of speech production and the manner of its production is of great importance in many occupations. For example, a waiter in public service cannot put his hand to the tracheostomy site if he has a tight collar and tie. Also, there is no question that the ordinary public that he serves would not fully sympathize with such a disability when they could not understand his speech and would conclude that the man is ill. Therefore, regardless of sympathy for the human problem, this would conflict with his job. While esophageal speakers in the laryngectomized can at times do extremely well, this is rare. Acceptable speech is attainable for 60 percent and that does not mean that it is adequate for the more demanding of occupations. Nor does it mean that the person can work in all environments, for example, in a coal mine or where there is danger of falling into water. Nor can he work in occupations where glottic closure is needed for heavy weight lifting. When we consider these factors, the penalty of a permanent tracheostomy is an economically staggering one for many.

Chapter 15 on *Neoglottic Reconstruction—the Staffieri Technique* states that the "goal of this group of surgical procedures is the development of a one-way, tracheopharyngeal fistula that permits the passage of pulmonary air in a manner that generates a vibratory airstream comparable to that produced by the normal larynx." However, in spite of the claim that this is a "Level 1," or most desirable solution, it would seem that any procedure that requires a permanent tracheostomy and fingertip closure for speech could hardly be called a most desirable goal. It may be satisfactory, but not a goal to shoot for. More of a problem in this type of procedure is the majority of cases done throughout the world who have an unacceptable degree of salivary aspiration. The procedure also has a problem of extreme hoarseness of voice that is notable even in the best neoglottis that can be created. In the article itself, 65 percent of patients are stated to have actively used the neoglottis for communication one year after the procedure. This compares to 50-60 percent of laryngectomized patients who use esophageal speech in all the surveys that we have been able to check on. This does not seem worth the dangers of aspirations for many of the patients that would otherwise have made attempts at neoglottis formation.

The method of reconstruction presented by Pearson, Hartman, and Woods in Chapter 14 for a T3 laryngeal carcinoma offered an ingenious tracheopharyngeal fistula for voice production utilizing uninvolved portions of the larynx. By preservation of the recurrent and superior laryngeal nerves on the uninvolved side of the larynx in satisfactory cases, a neoglottis is created for phonation. This is constricted during swallowing. The airway is maintained by a permanent tracheostomy. Thus, we still have the disadvantage of a permanent tracheostomy, but there are several advantages. The major advantage is an adequate fistula with which an unusually high percentage of patients succeed in producing good quality speech. An analysis of subglottic pressures by the authors showed that adequate levels for reasonable functions can be achieved in these cases.

The vertical partial laryngectomy as well as the horizontal or supraglottic partial laryngectomy would be preferred if a complete removal of all malignant tissues could be performed in this manner. When so possible, the secondary goal of "maximum preservation of the respiratory, phonatory, and sphincteric function of the larynx" can be achieved. This, of course, is the equivalent of a true, Level 1 goal. With no permanent tracheostomy or requirement of a finger for closure, we have a natural airway circumstance. This procedure can be done where there is up to one-half or more of the vertical dimension that must be removed, or, in the horizontal dimension, the excision of the superior one-half of the larynx with or without a portion of the base of the tongue or adjacent pharynx. Here it is worth restating that the "function preserved is function that does not require restoration."

Phonatory function is excellent in the majority of partial-laryngectomy procedures, but as stressed in Chapter 13 by Byron Bailey, "careful patient selection for this procedure is the key to a successful outcome in the majority of patients." The location and extent of tumor determines the appropriateness of the individual procedure.

No discussion of surgical-enhancement methods in the laryngeal patient can be concluded without mention of Dr. Singer's and Dr. Panje's method for plastic prosthetic devices between the trachea and esophagus. These devices are simple airway conductors from the trachea to the oral pharynx, though this methodology is still in a state of evaluation. However, they offer potential of good voice creation by simple reversible processes in a large percentage of cases. Complications can be noted in respect to aspiration of saliva, but much less often than with surgically created tracheoesophageal fistula. The voice is adequate in a large percentage of the cases in which the device has been used. The advantage, as stated, is in the ease of closure of the fistula by simply removing the device. The procedure must be done with the aid of a good speech teacher, and the care of cleaning of the device as well as its replacement must be taught carefully to a reasonably intelligent patient.

APPENDIX
Abstracts of Papers
Not Included in Full

SPEECH INTELLIGIBILITY AFTER LARYNGECTOMY—A REVIEW OF THE LITERATURE

ABSTRACT

Intelligibility after laryngectomy has been assessed by several researchers, but there has been little discussion concerning the reason for articulatory difficulty following laryngectomy.

In reviewing the literature of past studies of intelligibility after laryngectomy one finds great variability in the research design. Most of the studies were concerned with (1) consonant and vowel errors, and (2) phonemic category from most to least intelligible. Esophageal speech has received more attention than artificial larynx speech. The mean intelligibility scores were usually higher for the esophageal speakers than the artificial larynx speakers. Some of the discrepancies between the results of these studies were due to differences in the kinds of listeners evaluating the postlaryngectomees' speech.

Sally A. Bowman
Indiana University School of Medicine
Speech Clinic
1100 W. Michigan
Indianapolis, Indiana 46202

ACOUSTIC AND PERCEPTUAL ANALYSIS OF VOCAL DYSFUNCTION

ABSTRACT

There is a great need in phoniatric-logopedic diagnosis and treatment for objective criteria of vocal dysfunction. Today, voice analysis relies mainly on subjective visual and auditory observations. To make research methods for acoustical voice analysis clinically applicable, a project has been carried out in cooperation between the Institute of Logopedics and Phoniatrics at Huddinge University Hospital and the Speech Transmission Laboratories at the Royal Institute of Technology, Stockholm. Clinically experienced logopedists and phoniatricians evaluated 32 pathological and normal voices with respect to 26 perceptual variables on a 5-point scale concerning voice quality and pitch. A standard text (about 40 sec) was read by the subjects, and the signal was recorded on a two-channel tape recorder. The signal came from a spectacles-worn microphone with a constant mouth-to-microphone distance on one channel and on the other channel from a contact microphone put on the throat below the thyroid cartilage.

The evaluations of the voices were analyzed by factor analysis (Principal Component Analysis). The resulting factors were compared with acoustic measures from mainly three types of analysis: long-time average spectrum analysis (LTAS) and distribution analysis of the fundamental frequency, which was performed on the signal from the contact microphone. In order to analyze time-bound characteristics of the voice signal a frequency-perturbation measure was also used.

The results of the perceptual evaluation and of the acoustic measures were compared by means of multiple regression analysis.

This is a slightly revised version of a paper presented at the 9th International Congress of Phonetics, August 1979, Copenhagen.

Britta Hammarberg
Institute of Logopedics and
    Phoniatrics
Huddinge University Hospital
Stockholm, Sweden

Bjorn Fritzell
Institute of Logopedics and
    Phoniatrics
Huddinge University Hospital
Stockholm, Sweden

Lage Wedin
Institute of Psychology
Stockholm University
Stockholm, Sweden

Jan Gauffin
Speech Transmission Labora-
    tories at the Royal
    Institute of Technology
Stockholm, Sweden

Johan Sundberg
Speech Transmission Labora-
    tories at the Royal
    Institute of Technology
Stockholm, Sweden

REQUIREMENTS FOR DEVICES AND PROCEDURES AFTER TOTAL LARYNGECTOMY

ABSTRACT

This paper reviews the state of the art knowledge of laryngeal physiology and evaluates the parameters necessary for voice production following types of surgery for laryngeal cancer. Data from normal voice production as well as esophageal speech production are employed to identify certain relationships necessary to produce sound. Included are the relationships between esophageal pressure, subglottal pressure, and intraoral air pressure. The mechanical constraints of the neoglottis as a sound generator and the altered effect of the lips, teeth, and tongue as articulators will also be considered. Attention to the need for fistula, air by-pass, and other reconstructive procedures will be given.

Alternatives to current prosthetic devices and commonly used rehabilitation procedures will be discussed. The limiting factors for use of such devices and some requirements for their operation will be considered. Important is the manner in which various speech aids, types of speech, and surgical techniques can be evaluated for their communicative effectiveness.

Thomas Murry, Ph.D.
Veteran's Administration Medical Center
Audiology and Speech Pathology Service
3350 La Jolla Village Drive
San Diego, California 92161

312

A TWO-WAY CONVERSION OF THE WESTERN ELECTRIC #5 ARTIFICIAL LARYNX FOR INTRA-ORAL USE

ABSTRACT

Modifications of the Western Electric No. 5 electrolarynx are presented. These include a total conversion to an intraoral-type device with both the output transducer and the on-off switch mounted in a protective case remote from the main frame assembly. Assembly of the hand-held components and the modifications to the main frame are described and illustrated. Another modification includes conversion to a nine-volt battery for use by people who reside in remote areas where the #MN1604 battery is difficult to obtain. Dysarthric patients, using the intra-oral attachment described here or any other instrument may find it advantageous to provide multiple small holes in the mouth part of the intraoral tube to allow the escape of air when the end of the tube is occasionally blocked by the less than totally mobile tongue of the dysarthric patient.

Albert W. Knox, Ph.D.
Audiology and Speech Pathology Service
Kansas City Veterans Administration Medical Center
4801 Linwood
Kansas City, Missouri 64128

CONSIDERATIONS TOWARD THE DESIGN OF A TOTALLY AUTOMATIC ARTIFICIAL LARYNX

ABSTRACT

This paper establishes the need for the development of a self-activated artificial larynx for use with patients incapable of either esophageal voice or competent use of existing alaryngeal instruments. Contributions toward the development from other research and other disciplines is discussed and criteria are postulated for a prototype instrument. A block design of the instrument under development is presented with a list of solid-state components commercially available, that could contribute to the development. The projected development is postulated on several assumptions, among which are the adequacy of the VA-NU electronics package to provide the necessary input myoelectric potentials and the ability of discrete muscle movement or change in anatomical space to provide control of the continuous functions.

Albert W. Knox, Ph.D.
Audiology and Speech Pathology Service
Kansas City Veterans Administration Medical Center
4801 Linwood
Kansas City, Missouri 64128

INTRAORAL ELECTROLARYNX

ABSTRACT

The artificial electrolarynges currently available to the laryn-gectomy patient must be hand-held and either placed against the neck (Western Electric Electrolarynx No. 5) or held in front of the mouth (Cooper-Rand Electrolarynx). Patients who require such an instrument may react negatively to the need to hold them close to the face and the requirement that one hand be incapacitated while talking. Some laryngectomy patients resist using an instrument because of this and are therefore limited in their ability to communicate. Attempts to create a less-conspicuous but equally intelligible device have been reported and will be reviewed.

Since a concealed device that is easier to use was needed, a wireless, intraoral electrolarynx has been developed. This instru-ment consists of an earphone receiver and a pickup coil housed in the patient's denture. A separate transmitter with hand switch, worn under the patient's clothing, activates the receiver. An electronic receiver 1 mm thick is housed in the center of the denture, and the receiving coil surrounds the receiver. An Oticon® type AO 50 earphone weighing 10 gm was used for the speaker. The receiver/speaker enclosed in a denture was placed in the patient's mouth, and intensity readings of 64 db were obtained in an IAC booth (1405 ACT). The speaker was located in the buccal region at the point of the third molar, and a plastic tube attached to the earphone extended medially and slightly upward past the midline. The tube transmitted sound to the posterior region of the oral cavity to provide maximum resonance and prevented the tongue from occluding the speaker aperture. Two rechargeable batteries power the receiver/speaker for five continuous hours.

The transmitter is worn under the patient's clothing and consists of a single-turn, transmitting coil worn around the neck. This coil provides the mechanical support for the transmitter and batteries. The transmitter and batteries comprise a package measuring 65 × 35 × 17 mm and weighing 70 gm. Three batteries with a projected lifetime of six months supply the voltage to the transmitter.

Testing revealed that the instrument is not efficient when single-syllable words are spoken or when sentences contain fairly complex messages. However, the instrument is highly intelligible when everyday speech is communicated. The concealment of the device and its employment when the patient's hand is by his side are advantages not attributable to other electrolarynges. However, the sound produced by the intraoral electrolarynx is monotonic like other electrolarynges, and it is not possible to eat or drink with the instrument in place. Saliva may also occlude the plastic tube. Further research to eliminate these disadvantages is in progress.

Daniel Zwitman
The Center for Health Sciences
University of California
Los Angeles, California 90024

Siegfried Knorr
Department of Electrical Sciences
   and Engineering
University of California
Los Angeles, California 90024

SURGICAL ASPECTS AND PROBLEMS
WITH ARTIFICIAL LARYNX
OR ESOPHAGEAL SPEECH

ABSTRACT

The effects of various surgical procedures upon the production of speech in the laryngectomized patient are discussed. First, consideration is given to the traditional laryngectomy procedures where the voice is produced by air from the upper esophagus. This acts as the energy source for the substitute sound-generating area. The next technique discussed is that of the neoglottis directly utilizing the expiratory pulmonary airstream for sound production. The expiratory pulmonary airstream can also be shunted from the trachea to the hypopharynx or upper esophagus internally by surgically created tubes or externally by means of various devices. These artificial devices are either simple air shunts or they may contain vibratory components requiring varied surgical procedures for their creation. Finally, we consider vibratory, sound-producing electronic devices buried in the hypopharynx or dental plates.

Wilbur J. Gould, M.D.
Department of Otolaryngology
Lenox Hill Hospital
47 East 77th Street
New York, New York 10021

APPLICATIONS OF THE SONDHI TUBE IN SPEECH ASSISTANCE RESEARCH

ABSTRACT

The Sondhi tube, a one-dimensional acoustic transmission line with a characteristic impedance (reflectionless) termination, when properly constructed and calibrated, can have an output that is an approximation of the glottal sound-pressure wave. Such a device is useful, both as a nonresonant acoustic-measuring device and as a direct, real-time, glottal wave measuring device.

In my laboratories I have been using the Sondhi tube as a device for measuring the acoustic response of the electroacoustic transducers for the Texas laryngeal prosthesis system. By extension, this tube can be used to measure the acoustic output of many small devices without the usual worries about reflections and resonances.

As applied to humans, the Sondhi tube is being used, with auxiliary equipment and displays, to teach deaf persons to better control their speech pitch and volume.

Initial efforts are also being made to analyze the glottal wave of singers to determine what components of the wave are desirable and to assist the trainee to habitually form more desirable glottal waves.

R.L. Everett
Electrical Engineering Department
University of Houston
Houston, Texas 77004
318

INDEX